A BOOK THAT HAS TOUCHED CANADIANS FROM COAST TO COAST

"An absolutely riveting and wonderful book about a true story, a true life, *A Promise of Hope* is one of the best books I've read."

—Mary (Chomedey, Laval, QC)

"*A Promise of Hope* is an incredible family's tale of recovery, courage, faith, and conviction. A book worth reading, especially if your life has ever been touched by mental illness."

—Sarah (Conn, ON)

"I was hooked from the first paragraph. It is a beautiful tale of a woman's struggle with mental illness and her hope for recovery. A must-read."

—L. (Regina, SK)

"Autumn Stringam's *A Promise of Hope* is a page-turner, an exposé, a story of hope and courage, but mostly a story of love. It is an inside look at the suffering caused by bipolar disorder as well as the suffering caused by government officials, policies, and the powerful medical and pharmaceutical professions. Thank you for fighting for the rights of the mentally ill."

—Debra (Winnipeg, MB)

"It is fitting that this book is called *A Promise of Hope*; I am left inspired and confident."

—Sonja (Embrun, ON)

"All the chaos of bipolar disorder—the highs, the lows, the delusions, the anger, and the deep depression—are felt in a way that could never be accurately described by anyone who has not lived the story. Read it; you will be glad you did."

—Betty (Smithers, BC)

"*A Promise of Hope* by Autumn Stringam was one of the most mesmerizing autobiographies I have ever read. It was a quick read with a powerful message: there is hope for normalcy without resorting to drugs. A must-read for anyone interested in mental illness, especially bipolar disorder."

—Kathy (Aylesford, NS)

"A real page-turner from start to finish. This is a very moving book and one I will reread."

—Colleen (Daysland, AB)

"Autumn Stringam is definitely a very brave woman, not only for having overcome the challenges to her health and the obstacles of her legal battle, but also for writing so honestly about her experience."

—Alexandra (Waterloo, ON)

"This is one of the most powerful books I have read in a long, long time. I am so grateful to Autumn for having the strength to write it. I am happy she is a healthy person today."

—Gillian (Brampton, ON)

"Autumn Stringam shows herself to be a remarkable woman. She courageously lays a heartbreaking life out before the reader with faith that she may help those who have also endured bipolar disorder."

—Laurie (Bracebridge, ON)

"This book was absolutely riveting. I could not put it down. Autumn's journey was both heartbreaking and inspiring. Whether the supplement works or not, it offers hope that non-traditional approaches can offer help for those without hope."

—Laura (Grand Valley, ON)

A PROMISE OF HOPE

A PROMISE OF HOPE

AUTUMN STRINGAM

WITH AN AFTERWORD BY DR. CHARLES POPPER, M.D.

Collins

Published by Collins, an imprint of HarperCollins Publishers Ltd.

Originally published in trade paperback by Collins,
an imprint of HarperCollins Publishers Ltd: 2007
This trade paperback edition: 2009

An earlier, substantially different version of this work was
self-published by the author in 2006 under the title *These Painted Wings*.

The information contained in this book may not be applicable in any individual case.
Responsibility for any personal injury or other damage or loss arising from
the use or application of information in this book is expressly disclaimed.

HarperCollins books may be purchased for educational, business,
or sales promotional use through our Special Markets Department.

HarperCollins Publishers Ltd
2 Bloor Street East, 20th Floor
Toronto, Ontario, Canada
M4W 1A8

www.harpercollins.ca

Library and Archives Canada Cataloguing in Publication

Stringam, Autumn
A promise of hope : the astonishing true story of a woman
afflicted with bipolar disorder and the miraculous treatment that
cured her / Autumn Stringam; with an afterword by Charles Popper.

ISBN: 978-1-55468-509-7

1. Stringam, Autumn--Mental health. 2. Manic-depressive
illness--Alternative treatment. 3. Manic-depressive illness--Diet therapy.
4. Manic-depressive persons--Canada--Biography. 5. Coaldale
(Alta.)--Biography. I. Title.

RC516.S77 2009   362.196'8950092   C2008-908089-0

RRD 9 8 7

Printed and bound in Canada
Design by Sharon Kish

For my mother, Debora,
and the Shinah House she would have built.

INTRODUCTION

In the fall of 2007, my husband, Dana, and I and our four children set off from our home in Alberta in a camper trailer and drove all the way to the Atlantic Ocean to start our cross-Canada A Promise of Hope Tour 2007. We made it to Halifax just in time for the book launch and our first-ever live radio interview. Honestly, Dana and I have never been so nervous as we were when we walked into that studio. Terror and sheer joy combined to churn our stomachs in directions we never knew were possible. Later that day, Dana and I spoke to a small crowd at a local college auditorium. We shared our story and our hope for the prevention and resolution of mental illness for all those who suffer from it.

During the tour, we made new friends and met old ones again. Debra and her boy, now a healthy teen, came out to hear us in Halifax, Suzanne and Sabine in Ottawa, Sheila in Toronto, all with their spouses and all still healthy and blessed! Our friendships, first forged in our nation's capital on a day when defending our right to use nutrition over drugs for mental health seemed an impossible task, have blossomed. I basked in these friends' stories of continued recovery, of the growth of their families, and of the saving of their marriages because of their new-found health. The first two weeks marked a beautiful beginning to our cross-Canada tour and were a confirmation that what Dana and I were doing in trying to reach other families was a good thing and worth the effort.

But not everyone wanted to hear from us. Our beautiful beginning came to a screeching halt in northwestern Ontario. The press was small, the weather was terrible, and I was met with intense skepticism about EMPowerplus, the nutritional supplement that had healed me. I was stunned when some people said that we don't need a "miracle cure" for bipolar disorder. And, perhaps most surprisingly, I heard criticism of my mother and my grandfather.

It was a grim reminder of the continuing stigma of mental illness and the lack of understanding of it, something I hadn't experienced in a long time and certainly not in my world, where people know me and understand my recovery. By Thanksgiving, I was ready to give thanks for having a home to go to and to get there quickly. Were it not for my family's encouragement and good humour, the Promise of Hope Tour might have been the shortest cross-country junket ever!

The sun seemed to come out again over the Prairies. Events in Winnipeg, Regina, and a media visit in Calgary went well, and packed reading events on the West Coast were a beautiful ending and a wonderful lesson in patience and perseverance. As touching emails from readers poured in from all across Canada, I began to see the power of the written word. My story was changing hearts and opening minds to the possibility that a simple discovery made by laymen could actually be the undoing of a long tradition of sedation for the mentally ill. My story could be the beginning of a new understanding for people like me who wonder why they are sick and want desperately to find a way to real mental health. On the road home, Dana and I wrote down our memories, reviewing the journey we had chosen and my motivations for deciding to tell my story. It was a reminder of all the reasons I wanted to share my history with the world.

Of course, my first reason for writing *A Promise of Hope* and sharing my story was my children. Publishing my life story has opened the door to raw, honest conversation in our home. When strangers come to my door in tears, or a person stops me in the grocery store with a hug and a thank you, my kids can't help but overhear, can't help but begin to understand where I have been and how many others are still there, clamouring to climb out of the pit of depression or come down from the mountain of mania. And they are not ashamed. James, Samantha, Melanie, and Meagan are growing up able to talk about mental illness the way others talk about muscle aches or broken bones—painful but treatable, and possibly preventable.

When I consider the dark ages of medical intervention, I picture people like me locked up in filthy cells, beaten, or perishing from exposure or torture. Later on, as recently as the 1950s, the mentally ill would be lobotomized. Even today, most are medicated with harsh psychiatric drug combinations that rob them of thought and feeling. When I think of these forms of treatment, I see more clearly the blessings of my life and the age in which I was born. And I see more change coming.

I respect those who have gone before; acknowledging that the freedom, health, and goodness one enjoys is a result of another's sacrifice. I have respect and gratitude for the great pioneers of nutritional therapy, Dr. Linus Pauling and Dr. Abram Hoffer, whose work continues to breathe change and truth into mental health. This is confirmed by tens of thousands who have benefited from my father and David Hardy's discovery that broad-spectrum nutritional supplementation can resolve the symptoms of serious mental illness. On disappointing days I am buoyed by the hard work of Dr. Bonnie Kaplan, as well as the continued support of Dr. Charles Popper and others, including Dr. Scott Shannon, Dr. Estelle Goldstein, and Dr. Jonathan Wright. I am encouraged by the thirteen studies that are underway in universities the world over.

There is a cure for the chemistry of illness, but it is only through the love and support of those closest to me that I have found a cure for the pain of loss, the sorrow of stigma, and the habits of abuse that once plagued us. I'm happy to say that the cycle is broken. Curing the soul is the door to true recovery. True recovery begins with hope. May you find hope as you read through these pages of my life.

—Autumn Stringam
March 2009

I

When I look back now, through little-girl eyes, I see my mother moving in slow motion. At times my view is misty, like the view through a steamy window or a fine rain. She is young and tanned and heavenly. The breeze at her back pushes her thick dark ponytail to her cheeks in shiny, smooth wisps and waves. Her slim legs, full breasts, and rounded tummy speak of motherhood and God's grace—the kind of beauty you find only in a woman about to give life to another soul. Her face is flawless and radiant. Her wide eyes are separated by a low flat bridge, a small nose—Dad calls it a button nose. Her lips are soft; everything about her is soft.

Like the points of light that dance on her skin, light filters through the caragana bushes and fertile cottonwood trees that surround the garden. These branches, dressed in a playful throw of fresh green dewy leaves, filter the everyday from life, affording her the privacy and serenity that she loves to wrap around our home on the old acreage in southern Alberta.

It's Picture Butte, but Mom says it as Pitcher Beaut. I wonder why the place we live is named after a jug. And what's a beaut? I decide *beaut* is short for *beauty*, which is what this place is to me. And in my little-girl dreams, Mom is the centre of everything beautiful. I would do anything to stay near her side, near enough to touch any time I want to. She is the most beautiful thing in my life.

I sit on the edge of the garden, hunch-backed and cross-legged. My corduroy-covered bum is damp and cool in the grass, and my bare toes dig into the sponge of tossed soil. I am watching her as the sunlight plays over her body in flickers and flutters, highlighting her shoulders and knees, glinting off her hair and the round of her back when she stoops to bless the plants with her touch. Her mysterious hazel eyes shimmer in the shade of her face as she turns to speak.

"Now you be my little helper and pull out all the weeds."

"Yeah!" I hop up from my perch and tiptoe across the rows of fresh baby plants to rest at her side. I crouch, she kneels, and I watch as she shows me which small green living things to tear up by their roots. I am happy to be her helper. I know it makes her smile when I am doing something right. And her smile is a reward worth any price in my world. I work near her for a few moments, eager to do it right, like her. Mom leaves me to my job and wanders off down the row to tend to some other vegetable.

I crawl through the warm black soil to reach her and hold up my prize weeds. "Like this, Mom?"

"Autumn Dawn, those are pea plants, not weeds." She only calls me Autumn Dawn when I am in trouble—any other time, I am Dawny—yet her voice is still soft on the edges, and I like the sound of my full name on her lips.

She takes me by my empty hand and leads me back to the end of the row. I kneel next to her and watch her try to repair the damage. One by one she takes each plant from my fist, and with the hands of an artist, she tucks each broken stem and torn root back into the earth. Her fingers are long, a fine olive colour. The soft dirt is pressed under the bitten-down nails at the end of each fingertip as she gives the peas a second chance at life and us a second chance at a sweet fall salad.

I remember the first time I learned the merits of nail-biting.

"I have to bite them," she said to my daddy. "Clippers leave them too sharp, and I might hurt my little babies with them." Biting her nails was a habit she would not break. "For the sake of the children, Tony, for heaven's sake, the children." Blessed by heaven, the right thing to do. So I bit mine, too.

She was excusing a habit, but who could argue with her? Not Dad. She had a knowing glint, a silent laugh in her eyes, a flirtation, a mystery, a part of her that left me and him wanting more, wanting to be closer to her, wanting to give in to her, even when she didn't make sense. Dad knew better than to argue most times. Sometimes, when he did argue, it was just to let her win, just to watch her in victory. When Mom was winning, she was glorious.

I was born several weeks early because of the glory of Mom's winning, so the family story goes. She and Dad spent a rainy day playing cards in their tiny apartment. Mom kept winning. She was cheating, refusing to give up a card when it was called for. Game after game, Dad acted bewildered by her sudden luck in Go Fish. When she was finally caught, she laughed so hard that her water broke. Her memory of a card-playing triumph and a baffled and frustrated husband kept her giggling aloud for years afterward as she told the story I never got tired of hearing.

Once each of the pea plants is restored to its place in the ground, she relaxes. "Okay, so Dawny," she says with a breathtaking smile, white and smooth, "how about you and Angie go into the potato patch and work on your worm collections." I skip off to join Angie in the potatoes, with a glass Mason jar in one hand and a plastic sand shovel in the other. Weeds might look like peas and peas like weeds but worms are worms, and I know my worms.

Mom's baby belly stretched beyond her narrow hips, getting in the way of everyday things. It knocked against door frames and the backs of chairs, sopped water from the countertop at the kitchen sink, blocked our view when she stood near the television. It served as a plate rest for her and an oversized pillow for tired girls' heads. Especially for Sunni's.

Fluffy blonde Sunni truly was sunny as a two-year-old, but also quiet, thoughtful, and stubborn. She was the youngest of the three of us who loved to sit on the end of Mom's lap, each in turn gripping her belly as if we were starfish, holding on tight and pressing our faces into the top of it. The living thing inside would kick and thrash, making me shriek when the knots in her belly knocked against my hands.

One morning we came down the stairs to find a lady from church in our kitchen.

"Where's my mom?" Angie was the bold one among us.

"She went to hospital to have the baby," the lady said.

We danced and tore through the house, whooping and yelping. Another baby, another playmate, another sister. But no. When Mom came back there was no sister, just a tightly wrapped wiggly bundle. Fat and red with tufts of dark hair that would soon turn to the lightest blond, a stubby creature packed with endless energy, tight fists, and a bright toothless round grin. And a boy at that, our first brother.

"Babies aren't supposed to smile this early, Tony." Mom held her bundle snugly against her soft, flabby tummy.

"Well, that's my boy," said Dad. Dad, so young and fresh-faced, twenty-four years old. Married at eighteen and already a father to three daughters and a son.

Daniel was a lightning bolt, a supercharged battery mascot, packed full of mischief and masculinity—he was all-day entertainment on an acreage once dominated by girls.

The bathwater is fuzzy with bubbles—pink and blue oil slicks and tiny rainbows on fragile globes that dance on the water, foaming around the edges of our bent-up knees and arched backs and beach-ball bellies. With Angie behind me and Sunni nested in front, there is barely room in the tub for baby Daniel. He is always placed at the front of our bubble train, where Mom can reach him easily in case he slips on his soft bum and disappears beneath the foam. When the next baby is born, we will have to split the bathers into two groups. Four in a tub is already one too many.

"Where'd the soap go?" Mom wants to know.

Our hair is full of shampoo, lathered until the slippery mess of spice and flowers has filled our ears and allowed Mom to push the hair on each of our heads into an updo, stacked like stiff whipped cream on the tops of four portions of pink fruit.

"I feel it over here," Angie says. But as she presses the white Ivory bar to the bottom of the tub to grip it, the lump shoots to the surface, jetting into my back and then diving into the bubbles. It floats low in the water, now murky with the residue of garden and crushed leaves and chewed grass. "Oh, I lost it."

"Okay, so kiddos, let's play Find the Soap. I'll sing for you:

Where's the soap now? Where's the soap now?
Is it by my leg? Am I sitting on it?
Now it's here by Daniel, slipping back to Sunni,
Pick it up, pick it up."

All to the tune of "Are You Sleeping, Brother John?" Mom is our rock star. We laugh out loud, thrashing the water to cream, until finally Sunni grips the soft bar and raises it over her head, victorious. Large victories in small things fill our days with Mom.

Mom rinses the dessert topping from Daniel's silky baby head and pulls him out of the tub first, wrapping him in a thin hooded terry towel. The towel clings to his shoulders and sops the water from his white-blond flyaway hair. The hair is what we love best about our baby brother. Next year, as he learns to run, we will call him the White Streak.

Mom tucks Daniel onto her hip and goes to get us towels. She reaches into the wall nook behind the open door where the towels are neatly stacked. Dad has been tacking thin boards to the walls in a fancy V design, and the cedar makes its own perfume in the damp air. One wall is done, but the others are still naked and rough with plaster. The bathroom nook is torn open at the back, revealing the insulation and elderly studs.

"Get ready for rinsing, girls. See if you can help each other get the shampoo out of your— Ahhhhh!" All at once Mom is hysterical. "Get out, girls, get out right now. NOW!" But no, we are frozen. Is this a joke? A new game? We can't get out without our towels. If we drip on the floor, she gets angry.

"Get up, get out!" Mom holds Daniel off to the side on her hip and uses the other hand to wrench us up one by one, sloshing water onto the floor, soaking the bottom of her pants. Her strength is superhuman, and she moves faster than I have ever seen. Dragging three shiny, foamed, pastel bodies out of the bath and shoving us toward the door.

Sunni howls. Angie tries to push past Sunni to escape. This is no game; this is panic. I am voiceless until I see the reason for Mom's distress. On my way past the towels I peek into the guts of the walls. Two beads glowing in the shadows, two eyes set deep in the darkness. Blink, blink.

Now I howl, too, and run through the door into the parlour with its coal-burning stove. I dive face-first into the paisley couch. Even with my eyes shut and buried in a cushion, I can see those eyes in the wall. I can't burrow deep enough to escape them.

Mom wraps us in blankets and rinses our hair in the kitchen sink. The bathroom is off-limits. "Get here," she says into the phone. "It's a bat, Tony. . . . What time will you get here then? . . . I'll keep it locked in the bathroom, but you need to take care of this thing. The kids are freaked out, and I can't deal with it right now."

Dad arrives around suppertime.

"Is it still in the bathroom, Deb?"

"Yeah, we might as well eat before you go opening the door and letting that thing out."

"It smells great, hon," says Dad. Mom smiles for the first time since bathtime. When they are both smiling, I know everything will be all right.

Supper is pasta and bread and Taber corn. My favourite. Sweet butter and salty shakes over the pastel yellow.

I bite and squirt.

"Hey, Dawn's corn is spraying me." Angie is clear across the table, wiping at a thin line of milky corn juice in her hair and on her cheek. It's not entirely an accident.

"Careful, Dawny." Mom is distracted, caring for baby Daniel, stuffing his mouth with a mush of peas.

Squirt.

"Hey!"

The Taber corn made me forget the monster in the bathroom, but it did not forget us. It crept through the walls and found the hole in the kitchen wall, breaking free of its cedar prison. It came at us, a jagged blur. Screeching, flapping.

"The bat!" my mother screams. "Get it, Tony, get it!"

Screams of terror. We duck and bob and throw ourselves from the table as the bat flounders overhead.

"Get down!" Mom shrieks as the bat taps our heads and knocks on our plates. "Under the table." She's already hoarse as she hauls Daniel from his metal highchair. Plates crash, Taber corn splatters. Chairs skate and bounce and overturn, denting the walls.

Four children and one mom, wailing and diving. One dad laughing so hard he is weeping, unable to go after the bat, letting it get away. It escapes back into the deep caverns of fallen paper insulation and hollow wooden-slat walls.

The bathroom walls were very quickly finished, and Dad found all sorts of time to patch up other holes around the house. And life went on, our family happy.

Years later I awoke from a nap with a start, remembering the bat attack, the hysteria, the eyes, the laughter, everything so vivid I didn't know whether I'd dreamed the incident or lived it. I called Dad to ask.

We laughed again together, laughed so hard we cried.

"You were so little," he said. "I'm surprised you could remember it."

"I remember."

"Yeah, yeah, funny."

"So funny."

Both of us trailing off in the way a happy memory always winds down and peters out. Neither of us saying so, but both of us feeling it, each wanting to speak words to fill in the gaps for the other: I remember. I remember it wasn't all so bad.

Was it?

"Mom is crying again."

I look up from my place on the living room floor to see Angie standing above me. Yesterday's pigtails are still in her shoulder-length hair. Sleeping on them has pulled up a fine halo of fluff, rising from her centre part and bunching over the elastics by her ears. Angie is whispering, so I know this is important. It is Angie's job to keep track of how Mom is feeling and to make Mom okay. It is my job to take my cues from Angie and do what she tells me to do when Mom needs our help.

I get up from the floor, dropping Raggedy Ann and Andy onto the speckled carpet. Mom has left us to care for ourselves, and I am perfectly happy here on the floor in the living room, but . . .

Angie needs me. She hauls me by the arm and I stumble across the warm shag onto the grainy hardwood. My bare feet pick up bits of lint and dirt as I shuffle to keep up. We pass the stairs and creep around the fuzzy paisley couch. I see Mom. She is in a heap, lying on her side with her head on the armrest. Her back is curved and her hands are tucked between her knees. Maybe she is just getting warm by the stove, but no, the stove is cold. I want to go back to the Raggedys, but Angie won't let go of my arm.

I startle a little as Mom shakes and heaves with a silent sob. I can see her tear-stained cheeks, but not her eyes. Her hair has slumped over her forehead, a shroud for her tears. I don't like this. Angie gives me the look: We have to do something.

Maybe if we make her talk, she will remember us.

"Mom, can we have some lunch?" It is all I can think to say.

She answers with a sob and a deep, woeful sigh. I crouch low to her chest. Angie stands close to Mom's head and pats her on the top of her round shoulder. Mom shrugs Angie's hand off. She is awake. I need her to speak. I need her to be okay. This is scaring me.

I lean in close. She doesn't smell okay. Her usual scent of hair conditioner and baby powder mingled with Tide laundry detergent is gone. Now she wears a nippy smell of unwashed hair and a greasy pillowcase. I draw back a bit.

"Mom?"

"Go get some pretzels from the cupboard," she says. She pushes her hair across her brow with the back of her hand—just enough for me to see her puffed and swollen eyes. Her black eye makeup is flaking onto her high cheekbones, and her lashes are dark and clumpy and wet. Her nose is shiny and her normally smooth olive cheeks are sallow, streaked, and blotched with red. A few long hairs are stuck to the side of her damp face. I don't like the way she looks. I need to get away from her.

"Pretzels, yum!" Angie and I escape to the kitchen and ransack it for snacks.

Before long, Dad comes home.

"How come you're home so early, Daddy?" Angie and I run to meet him as he pushes through the cluttered doorway. I am so relieved.

"Where's Mom?"

"Mom's crying, Dad. You should help her stop crying." Bold Angie pushes him toward Mom.

"I know Mom is sad, girls." He kicks off his shoes and sets down his metal lunch box. "Grandpa is sick, and we have to go see him right away."

They dropped us off with neighbours while they went off. They came back for a day and then left again. The second trip was for the funeral. We didn't get to go; Mom said a funeral wasn't a place for children.

"Why did he die?" I asked on a day when Mom wasn't crying.

"He ate too much salt and his heart stopped working."

She got worse after that, spending most of her days on the couch. She didn't get dressed. Sunni and Daniel were toddlers, aged three and one. If Mom got up, it was only to do something for them. Angie and

I were big girls, six and five. We didn't need Mom's help. But we did need her.

"Mom, it's time to get up. Puleeese, puleeese, will you get up?"

"Leave me alone, Dawny," Mom would say low, mumbling under her breath.

I would do anything to be near her. So would Dad.

"What are you doing?" I ask. Mom is on the couch, and Dad has a bunch of shiny tools and cloths and a little board that looks like sandpaper. Mom's foot is in his lap and he is fussing over her toenails.

"Oh, Dad is fixing my feet because I can't reach them." Her latest baby belly won't let her bend that far.

"Can I do it, too?" I ask Dad.

"Yup, you can rub this on Mom's heels so they won't crack any more." Dad gives me a squirt of perfumed cream and I rub it into the cracks of Mom's rough heels. Her feet are dark on the bottom and white around the edges and her toenails are grey. I decide that I don't want to touch them after all, but Dad seems to love every minute of touching her.

After a while I begin to love it, too.

"Your mom is a queen," Dad says. She purses her lips and flutters her dark lashes at him. When he has finished, he gathers the cloths and tools and leans over to give her a kiss on the forehead. She closes her eyes as he kisses her. I want the moment to last forever.

Mom's time on the couch stretched from days to months. Our world was not okay without her in it. Angie and I tried everything to include her in our play, anything to draw her out of her world and into ours. We'd pull her long locks over the soft armrest of the couch and play hairdresser, trying to put her hair in braids and fancy knots. Angie would work on one side and I on the other. Sometimes Sunni would join us, and we would get our combs and brushes locked together under the dark brown thickness of Mom's hair.

"Ouch! Back off." We would drop the combs and brushes and let her sort out the tangled mess. She'd lie down again and let us start all over.

"Girls, you need to help Mom with the babies," Dad said as he left for work in the morning. Angie and I tried, but there were a lot of scratched faces and fistfights and tug-of-wars over babies and toys and doll clothes.

When we needed her to leap into action, Mom was slow and sorrowful. Most of the sunshine had gone out of our house.

Mom gave birth to sweet baby Bradford in the heat of the summer. His dark curls and olive skin made his bright blue eyes look like glass. He was precious and soft, and he didn't thrash around as much as Little Daniel, the White Streak. Baby Brad had the softest ears, downy and pliable, kissable, suckable. Mom would kiss his face and slide her mouth over his hair. Then, making the softest pecking sound, she would nibble his ears with her dewy lips. Brad was a cuddler, and Mom loved to cuddle her second son. Her father was dead, but she said he had appeared to her in the delivery room. She was consoled by his presence at the birth—and for a time life felt the way I wanted it to feel.

I try to remember all the good things. Our home once boarded teachers who worked across the gravel moat that separated our land from the old school. Now the school was a community hall used for Christmas pageants and the like. To the south was a tiny corner store—the place to buy Popsicles and Pep chocolate mints. Just a sprint through the garden, then across the broad plank bridge that spanned the wet ditch without rails or sides, then over the gravel road and we were there. To the north ran the long driveway that ended in the garage, a building that was much newer than the house and the barn. The faded barn stood off in the farthest corner of the horses' field, gated by barbed wire, shaded by trees and overgrown bushes. It sagged and creaked and grinned at me like an old man with a wide smile. It was a house for mice and ants and our mare and her wild colt that Dad named Diablo.

Inside the house a macramé square hung, its wooden beads and pottery bits interwoven in an earthy design. Blue and teal peacocks clung to the bathroom wall. They were made of wire and clay—glossy and misty in the steam of our bath. I remember other things—the dry wooden floorboards, the long shaggy carpet, the table with chrome edges and sparkles embedded in its creamy smooth Formica top; the tall, brushed stainless steel pedestal that stood in the corner of the living room beside the couch, domed with tinted plastic to protect the record player. The speakers were round balls that sat in cups on the floor anchored to the pedestal with fine black wire. We weren't allowed to roll them about. And I remember the tunes of the Beatles, the Monkees, and America. They were Mom's favourites. She played "Sister Golden Hair" the most.

At night, after Daddy was home and the dishes were done, we were tucked in our beds. I often fell asleep to the sound of the silver record player—the melodies and rhythms that sounded through the floorboards and into my mattress. The life that Mom and Dad lived after bedtime was a mystery to me. There was laughter and music, the smell of good food, whispers in the dark stairwell just outside my room, and creaks across the floor on their way to bed.

"I have to pee," I whisper to Angie.

"Me, too."

"Should I yell to Mom?" No. Mom had already tucked us in twice after the I'm hungry and I need a drink ploys.

"I'm going in the upstairs bathroom," Angie says. She disappears into the dark, and I creep to the top of the stairs. The music carries up from the living room, up the stairwell to me. Another of Mom's favourites is playing: "A Horse with No Name."

I want to sing along, but I can't get caught sneaking down the stairs to the bathroom. I grip the rail as I tiptoe down the first flight. I stop on the landing to look out over the yard. The horses are kneeling, asleep under a lumpy, bumpy, thick-barked saggy tree that looks like a frumpy old woman in the corner of the field. Its branches are low and broad, arcing from the ground into the sky. I giant-step over the one squeaky stair tread and patter down the rest. At the bottom I feel the breeze from under the front door against my ankles. The bathroom is the other way, but I can't help it. I must steal a peek into the living room. I hold the edge of the wall, the wooden frame of the arched entry. I lean in to see.

There they are. Barefoot, toes deep in the shag carpet. Woven into each other, swaying. Mom's face is on Dad's shoulder. His face and his hands are in her hair. Her arms are loose over him, fingers caressing his neck at the top of his collar. My heart beats fast for them. I feel warmth over my whole body, thrilled down to the chill of the floor. So this is their secret life, the after-hours affair that is only for them.

The music stops. They don't. They hold each other, swaying still, until the next song begins. Mom shifts her head and I think she might see me. Then sleepily she turns back as Dad pulls her around for a kiss, warm and deep. She sinks into his lips and I feel a blush on my cheeks. I'm not supposed to be watching a kiss like this. I turn away and grip my pyjamas above the knees, picking my way back up the stairs.

I don't have to pee after all. I lie in bed, comfortable, secure, glad for them, glad for me. This is life as it should be. This is music with a new meaning. From now on when I lie in bed and feel the music through the floor, I will see it, too, in that dance. It is the best sound I will ever see: a lullaby, a kiss good night, a security blanket, a promise.

Spring came again to our little acreage. Snow gave way to patches of brown, which gave way in turn to the glory of green. The trees sprouted sappy leaves and robins' nests, and the yellow-breasted meadowlarks topped the fence posts and warbled at the sky. Long field grasses filled out the landscape and made soft cool beds for us in the shady spots.

We played in the shelter of the trees and bushes. The spring wind whipped through the branches. I loved the feel of it, clean and cool off the Rockies, thrashing about in my fine hair—whipping locks of blonde and brown into my face and mouth, sticking strands to the damp beneath my nose. I loved the sound of it, too—a rushing, hushing, shushing of the wind through trees. It filled me with awe, the size of the sound, enough to make me want to whisper, as if we were in church.

The earlier dawn of each day beckoned us to play out among the dogs and the chickens, the horses, and, briefly, the goat.

Baby Brad, my mother's fifth child, was allergic to cow's milk, so Dad bought the goat for its milk, not a gift she gave willingly. Or ever. On her first day in the family Mom named her Nanny Goat. Nanny tore down our fence and broke her leash. She ran away. She climbed on the roof of our station wagon, denting the hood and scratching the paint.

On her second day Mom began calling her Damned Nanny Goat. Damned Nanny kicked and charged when Dad would try to milk her. She spent her third day on the acreage butting the dogs and terrorizing the children. On her fourth day Damned Nanny was out of the family, and baby Brad was getting his goat's milk in cartons from the market.

Grandpa's death seemed long past to me, but on the first anniversary the scab on Mom's heart was torn off, and she was back on the couch. Brad was now crawling and busy, needing her attention, too. On this anniversary, rather than being merely sore and sad and vulnerable, she was agitated and sleep deprived and broken.

"Hurry and eat your breakfast." Mom hovers over us with a rag, waiting to wipe down the table. We can't shovel the food in fast enough to suit her.

"Awww, I don't want oatmeal, it makes me hot." I slouch in my chair and kick the metal legs. Ting-ting-ting.

"This isn't a restaurant, Dawny. If you don't like it, you can make your own damned breakfast."

Her tone hurts me. My nose stings. I won't cry. But why is she so mean? I pack in the oatmeal. I sweat. I wish she'd go back to the way she used to be.

Mom clears up and washes the babies' faces. She marches all of us up the stairs to the girls' room.

"Okay, so I have your clothes laid out here," she says. "Today we are wearing our nice play clothes." Our bed is a double mattress that lies flat on the floor. She has already tucked the blanket under the corners, fluffed our pillows, and put our clothes out in piles. Angie, Dawny, Sunni, Daniel, and Brad—all line up ready to be dressed.

"Where are we going?" I ask.

"Nowhere."

"Then why are we getting dressed?" Usually when Mom is sad, we can stay in our pyjamas all day.

"Because Auntie Colleen and Cousin Melanie are coming over."

"Yahoo!" Melanie. I love Melanie. I dance on the mattress, but Mom grabs my arm and sits me down and yanks a T-shirt over my head so hard my ears burn. What did I do?

When all of us are dressed, Mom herds us back down the stairs and sets us to work picking up strewn toys. We finish just as we hear Aunt Colleen's truck crunching gravel in the driveway.

Mel and I lounge on the lawn, picking at the fresh green grass. If a blade is pulled up just right, it leaves a sweet, soft, white tip to chew on.

Mel has such a bright smile. She pushes her tongue up to her teeth when she laughs, and her dimples are the prettiest things I have ever seen. Some nights I lie in bed, boring my fingers into my cheeks, hoping that in the morning I will have dimples like hers. I like the sparkle on Mel's clean blonde hair. She is so pretty and so tidy. She always has colourful bows in her hair and clean clothes. I try not to notice my own hand-me-down T-shirt, worn-out shorts, and grimy fingernails bitten down.

Mel spits out a chewed stalk of grass. "Do you think that we can get an ice cream?"

"I hope so." But I won't dare ask. The talk in the house is loud, urgent, angry.

"Vanilla?"

"My favourite." I'm thinking Mel might get away with asking. She is so cute and she is company. But the talk inside spills out the open windows, so it's not safe to ask now. I say my thoughts aloud. "My mom is mad."

"My mom is mad, too." She gives me the drift of what we're hearing from inside the house. "Grandma has a boyfriend. He's really mean, and now Uncle Gordy and Uncle Bruce have to live somewhere else." She always knows so much of the adult stuff about the family.

Mom's two brothers were the youngest of eight kids in her family. Gordy was in his early teens, the youngest child born to Grandma. Bruce was adopted and a few years younger.

The voices carry out onto the lawn.

"They need me, Colleen, it's just what Dad would want me to do."

"De-bor-a, you have five kids already. You can't take on two big boys. It's crazy." Aunt Colleen speaks with a lisp and a hint of sarcasm that makes me grin. I think she is smart. She says Mom can't help her brothers. That she shouldn't even try.

"I'm talking to Tony when he gets home." I hear it in that voice of hers. Mom will win this debate. She always wins.

One Saturday soon after, Mom and Dad brought garbage bags, a broom, and some rags from the kitchen. They climbed the stairs and we followed. A mystery was about to be unveiled. They were about to open the locked door on the upstairs landing.

The room was much less mysterious than my imaginings. It smelled of rot and dust and filth. We cleared out cobwebs and rodents' nests and stacks of papers and boxes of useless broken trinkets. Under that we found dirty plaster and a floor strewn with mouse dung and more dust. We found no treasures here. And within hours I took sick.

My eyes swelled shut, and I developed lumps behind my neck and in my chest, groin, and knees. I became feverish, going from sweats to chills. My nose ran. I was on fire. I stayed sick for days. Then the coughing began.

They said I was hypersensitive. Whatever it was, it began the day we cleaned out a filthy place and let Gordy and Bruce into our home.

Mom welcomed them with open arms. She thought they might help her with chores and childcare. Bruce did play with us. He loved to take Angie and me on dirt-bike rides through the garden paths. He was kind to the dogs and he helped when Mom asked. Having Bruce around was like having an older brother—I just loved him.

Not Gordy. He left us after only a few weeks, and I was glad. Gordy was old enough to babysit. That freed Mom for shopping and church functions. He didn't play with us, except to tease and make fun. He amused himself by agitating us. Being around him always ended in anger and shame. Gordy was thick and stocky, his dense hair and deep-set eyes spaced wide by a low, flat bridge. His mouth was full of straight teeth covered by lips so full they looked inside-out to me. His hands were beef steaks with fat sausage fingers.

One night he is left in charge. I cry when Mom gets ready to leave. She tells me to shush, that she will be home soon after I go to sleep. I don't usually cry when she leaves, but this time I can't stop myself.

We are already bathed and dressed for bed before Mom leaves. When it is time for sleep, Gordy shoos us up the stairs.

"Take off your panties," Gordy says. "It's time for bed."

"I wear my panties to bed."

"No, your mom said you had to take off your panties tonight." Gordy glares at me. Mom said I had to listen to him. So I slip my panties off, careful not to show my bum.

"Hey," says Gordy, "I saw you standing on your head on the couch today. Do you think that you can do it against the wall? It's pretty tough to do. Do you think you are big enough?"

I hate his voice. It has a sly, cutting edge. I feel as if bugs are crawling inside my clothes when he teases. But what I hate more is the voice Gordy uses when he tries to get me to do favours for him. "Dawny, would you go get me a cup of water?" He whines and grins sideways when he asks. Now he is using both voices. But he's wrong about one thing.

"I can stand on my head anyplace."

"Yeah? I don't think you can do it against this wall. You're probably not big enough. Still a baby."

"I'm no baby. I'm six." I go to the wall and put my head down. My hair is damp against the floor. I place my hands out a ways from my face and peek through my legs. I see Gordy upside down though my ankles. He rises from the end of the mattress and comes at me. His sandy hair, so thick that it cannot lie flat, sticks over his ears. His face is blotchy red, his smile sticky and nervous. He licks his fat lips.

"Go on, you little baby, let's see how long you can stay up."

I spread my legs on the wall for balance. I am not a baby. I can do this—

Gordy is over me. He grips my ankles against the wall. A surge of heat and pressure and confusion rip through me.

It's hard to breathe. I choke and . . .

I sit bolt upright in my bed. Angie rises to join me. The room is black. There are no sounds, only my retching. Vomit has filled the hollows of my eyes and ears. It's in my hair.

"Mo-o-om," Angie cries out. Her voice is raspy with sleep. "Mo-o-om," she wails as she tries to get away from me and the smell of me. She rolls onto the floor.

"Oh, crap," Mom says as she pushes through the door. "Tony, you'd better get in here."

Dad bursts in. I am awake now, my throat burning.

I raise a howl.

"Hush," says Mom. "Don't wake the babies." She isn't angry, but she will be if I wake them up. Pyjamas, sheets, quilts—she strips away the layers of bedding and clothing as Dad takes me.

The bath is warm. As Dad dumps the bucket over my head and scrubs and rinses, I see bits of curvy pasta and corn and chunks of hamburger bobbing on the water. I'm fascinated as the bits float awhile, then sink around my knees. I'm exhausted and spooked by a feeling in my head. Even bathing in my vomit doesn't bother me.

"I can't remember anything, Daddy."

"That's okay, Dawny, you're tired." He wraps me in one towel and dries my hair briskly with another.

He's right, I am tired. That's all. He scoots me back up the stairs to the bedroom where Mom has opened the window. She dresses me in panties and fresh pyjamas and tucks me back between clean sheets. Then she arranges my damp hair away from my face.

"Are you okay?"

"I can't remember anything."

"What?"

"I can't remember last night." I want to tell her how much this scares me. About the empty feeling, the panic. I want to tell her how something is not right in my head. But I am only six. I can't find words big enough to say.

"You're fine. You're just sleepy. Both of you get back to sleep—love ya, see you in the morning." Her dry feet scuff across the floor. She slips out, leaving us in the dark.

I can't close my eyes. I am nervous still.

"Angie, are you awake?"

"Yup."

"Do you want to play hairdresser?"

"No."

"Will you draw on my back?"

"No, you draw on my back." I reach out and touch Angie's back. With my pointer finger, I draw a house, then a dog, then a car and a letter A.

"I can't remember last night," I whisper. "I don't know how I got in bed." Angie doesn't answer. Her breathing is deep and calm and rhythmic. She was asleep before I got to the letter A.

I lie awake for a long time. I strain to remember the night. I know the day just fine. Angie and Sunni and I went shirtless into the horse's field.

The sun was hot and dry. The field was flooded with irrigation water, cool and fresh. We used the flat grass as a slide. We ran and dove on our bellies and slid into the water like otters. I remember supper, the pasta and bread and meat sauce. There was the fight in the living room over who would piggyback Dad first. Then . . . nothing.

The void is deep and dark. Odd, though, it isn't lonely. I have company in this dark place.

It is the very first time she comes to me. I feel her with me—not beside me, but inside my body, inside my head, a girl at the back of my brain. I am curious about her, not afraid. She doesn't speak, and neither do I. She doesn't startle me. She is just there, waiting. She feels natural and necessary. She comforts me.

I step back into my mind to take a closer look at her, this girl back there. She has no face, no body. For now, she has no voice. Even so, I know she is beautiful. She is my friend. Her presence is new but familiar, like a worn, warm sweater when I put it on to cut the chill on the eve of the first fall frost.

I don't ask why she is there; I just know I need her. I spend the night in silence with her, two friends dressed in matching sweaters. I need her, and she is there for me: My Girl. I drift off to sleep just as the sun pokes over a patch of gold on a distant farmer's field.

4

Gordy is such a small part of my memory of the acreage home. He's like a Waldo lost and never looked for, never even asked about on the immense detailed landscape of my mind. A busy and mostly benign landscape of memories it is, too, the acreage. Shades of pink and blue scribbled on packing paper, crayons scattered over the tabletop, magnets on the fridge, rainbows and dogs. Pokey, the shaggy collie mix who bit tires as a diversion and licked my face as much to lap food as bestow his love. Tawny, the mutt with a snake's lanky, bendy body and short, yellow hair. Tawny was a nervous thing with crusty eyes who trembled like an electric massager as he slept, muffled in a heap of blankets at the end of my bed. Goats, pigs, horses. Kids, oh yes, lots of kids, mostly my own brothers and sisters. Ice cream cones and mousetraps, a shared mattress, a dusty wooden floor, and a deep shaggy carpet in the living room.

That shag. Mom always had to have shag. It meant something to her. Maybe it was the one tangle in her life she felt she could handle, something she could survey and measure and fix at a stroke. She'd had an extra long shag carpet in her first home with Dad, the kind that needed to be raked daily into standing straight or else it was a shameful mess.

Left too long, shag showed all the traffic patterns and lay in a random chaotic mess. Left alone, even a clean shag looked dirty.

After she had finished grooming the carpet, she would tiptoe around the edges to avoid wrecking a masterpiece of order, a single level spot in a life of so many ups and downs, a tended, temporary state of peace like a Japanese garden of stones. Raked into shape, even a dirty shag looked clean.

On the practical side, shag was a great place for kids to play, soft and warm in a chilly home, like a blanket for toes and a mattress for bony bums. I used to dream of owning the acreage again. Now I just dream of a house with shag carpet. It's a rare find now, but every time I walk on shag, I have to fight the urge to pull off my shoes and go barefoot.

Shag. The woolly mammoth look and feel of it takes me back to Picture Butte, the only place I ever long for, the only time I wish to return to. If only we had stayed there. We should have lived there forever. None of the other things would have happened. Or so I like to think.

Dad. At the very top of the acreage memory is a picture of my father, muscular and lean, brown hair pushed off to one side, his angular face and masculine chin resting on a bare forearm. So young and so intense, he is sitting, slouching, fidgeting, reckoning, pestering numbers—poring over an engineering problem. His books are spread across the table-top, each graph and chart and math table a window. Each of them gives him a peek at some part of his solution, daring him to put the fragments into a single coherent picture.

His absolute absorption in the problem renders him oblivious to his children and our chaos around him. We can shriek and wail and argue and never faze him. We can run pell-mell like a dust devil across the great Alberta plain, and he will not look away from his calculus. Oh, the racket it takes to pull his attention away from those books and into the kitchen, to find us standing at his side, waiting. When he blinks twice and focuses on us, it is as if he is awakening from a slumber so deep and entrancing, it has made him forget where he was when he went to sleep.

We wait for him to remember, wondering how he may react to each new awakening.

Will he tell us to be quiet, although he never even heard our noise until we cried to him like an out-of-tune chorus in a band?

Or maybe give that deep grumble in his chest, roll his eyes, and glide back to his work? No more, kids. No more.

Or take an otter's dive onto the floor to tickle and wrestle and hug our breath away until we have shrieked and laughed ourselves into exhaustion and find ourselves sedate enough for bed, letting him get back to pestering his engineering problem?

We risk a huge letdown if he dives back into the books instead of to the floor. But it is worth that risk, even if he slides off his chair only once in a great while.

I remember how he looks while I stand there at his chair waiting and hoping. He is tough, intent, focused. He is reserved, except for his eyes. They are guileless, like a puppy's, and the deepest blue. He is filled with goodness, humour, and sincerity. He is the strength in our home, a rock when we need a place to anchor us and a soft place for Mom to land when she is falling apart.

I learn to love learning by watching my dad. He is the smartest man I know. He makes me want to know all the secrets he has discovered at the kitchen table. If I study, if I pour myself into my grade one reader as he does into his thick books of numbers, I might know what he knows. I want to be him, but I cannot. I want to be like him, but I am not. This I know and dread above all other things, even as a barely aware child: I am like my mother.

"Daddy is writing an exam today, so when he gets home, we want to have all the toys picked up and a special supper for him," she says.

"What's an exam?"

"It's a test to see if he remembers all the math he has been learning in the nighttime." Mom fidgets with her fingers, picking at her nails and biting them as she busies herself in the kitchen. I can see that this test means as much to her as to him.

So it means a lot to me, too. "Will he remember?"

Mom stops. With the back of her damp hand, webbed with suds, she brushes the stray hair from her face, sweeping it back toward the ponytail at the base of her neck. "Your dad is so smart and works so hard. He'll remember what he learned, and we'll all be so happy when he is done." She is so proud of him. She smiles when she talks like this. She loves him so.

I want that. I want her to say those things about me. So I need to be smart like Daddy. I am trying hard. Some days I think it is working. Every morning Angie and I dress and run to the yellow school bus. Most mornings Mom stands and waves in the door. She blows kisses and calls to us to be good and remember that she loves us. Sometimes, when we come home, she greets us with a call from the kitchen. I hear her singing; I smell cookies. When I see her, she smiles. On days like this Mom is okay, and I am okay.

But not every day is like this, and I know I need to try harder. I must be like Dad. I must.

He did remember his math. After the exam he found a new and better job as a boiler engineer for a prison in the town of Peace River. We moved farther north into Alberta, a fourteen-hour drive north, to the edge of the Peace—to me, it was the edge of the world.

5

Our home in the Peace Country was one of a row, lined up like Monopoly properties, straight and perfectly spaced on a hilltop overlooking the prison. It was winter—the bitter northern February of 1980. The small split-level house lacked character. Identical except in colour to every other house on the row, it was boxy and tight and boring.

The front window overlooked the narrow asphalt road and a slope angling down to a highway. It was on this hill that we first enjoyed real sledding on a mattress of powder, deep, white, and dry—not crusted like the wind-swept mounds of southern Alberta. The broad slope ended in a curve up toward the road. The curled slope braked our slide in a *shush* and *whoof* of powder and ice crystals. Again and again we took the flight on our wooden sleigh, until our fingers were numb and our toes burned. Then, with chapped cheeks and frozen nostrils, we would clamber back up the slope to the house.

But too soon the postcard winter became too much of a good thing. The sequined snow bedeviled the Peace Country. For eight months out of the year the rolling tundra wore either its eye-aching white crunch or the heart-aching brown sludge of the melt. Then came a sudden heat and the bugs of summer like the plague on pharaoh. Mom could find no peace in the Peace Country. Close neighbours and sheer curtains exposed us in our play. Unlike on the acreage, people here could hear our shrieks and wails.

"Be quiet!" Mom would hiss. We had more kids than any other family in the row of houses, and Dad worked at the jail with all the other dads on that street. She didn't want the ladies talking about her unruly, obnoxious children. She didn't want us to embarrass Dad. She was pregnant again. She knew that the sight of her, waddling with her round belly, a train of five eager ducklings trailing after her, made the neighbours laugh.

"Don't make a scene, please," Mom would beg us as we pulled into the grocery store lot. "The first one to yell in the store is getting a spanking when we get home." We tried to obey. But inevitably Sunni would pinch Brad, or I would step on Angie's heel, or Daniel would make a grab for the cookies on the shelf and then freak out when Mom snatched them away. There was always a cry for help. There was always a scene. Always.

Then, too, the cashier would count us, pointing her finger at each one of us as we filed into the checkout to pay for the cart filled to the top with groceries.

"Are all of these your children?"

"Yes." Mom would put on the mask of a proud smile. "I guess I finally figured out how it goes."

"Oh?"

"We won't be having any more."

"Oh." The cashier would laugh. Mom would force her grin. She knew. They thought her foolish to be pregnant again. They thought her silly and uneducated and out of control. She was not proud. She was not happy. This was not her dream. At least not every day.

As the summer sun finally dried out the Peace Country, another baby boy came into our lives. Mom was thrilled with him. Baby Joseph, with his dark blue round eyes and chocolate hair, belonged in a Renaissance painting, a cherub in the arms of a noblewoman, an angel hovering near the Madonna's shoulder.

"He reminds me of my dad. He's so handsome," Mom gushed when her new friends came to visit.

Mom wasn't the only one who was charmed by Joey. Even when he was only a few days old, his quick gassy grin and meaty legs thrilled the rest of us kids. He made us laugh. He made us want to play house with him as if he were one of our toys. He was everyone's baby.

Until one day when Mom and Joey disappeared to the bedroom

upstairs to stay. The excitement of the new baby was over, and Mom was too tired for the rest of us, too dark to endure the day. There were a few weeks left before school would begin, and they were as slow in passing as the days before Christmas. One after the other, each one longer than yesterday, the days dragged. Without Mom, the house was dark, and nothing could light it up. She spent all her mornings and afternoons with Joey, tucked away up the stairs in her bedroom. And we, bored and lazy, stayed downstairs. We watched television and ate peanut butter and sticky peach jam—sometimes on bread, sometimes not—and waited for the morning when she would descend the stairs and sing to us again.

We entertained ourselves by ripping at each other's hair, ganging up on one another, rampaging through the house. Ear-piercing screams for help might bring her out of her solitude. But we never knew which mom it would be. Angry Mom? Or Dark Mom?

Would she rage at us for the mess? Send the little ones off to corners and make me and Angie help her clean up, all the while muttering to herself about how ungrateful and ill-behaved we were? Sometimes it was a relief to see that mom. It was better than the mom who slumped down the stairs to take in the destruction with dull hooded eyes, her shoulders rounding toward her chest, her belly slumping forward over her hips. This mom did not talk, let alone sing. Her empty eyes said she might never sing again.

6

"Arrgh, I'm so bored." Angie is on the floor of the living room, and I am drawn into a ball on the end of the couch. There is nothing on TV today, no one to play with but each other. Sunni, Daniel, and Bradford are nearby, each absorbed in boredom and mischief by turns. At eight and seven years old, Angie and I are poor babysitters. Crusted cereal bowls lie about the floor. Spoons, too, tongue-smeared peach and brown. And crusts of peanut butter and jelly sandwiches.

Little Daniel is yelling in the kitchen. "No! No! No!" He's in a panic, getting punched and pulled, but I am not moved. I know already by the sound that this one will get out of control. Maybe that will bring Mom—one of her—down the stairs. I want it to get out of control. I want to see her.

"It's mine!"

"No, MINE!"

Sunni, Daniel, and Brad are battling it out in the kitchen over who knows what. Angie and I trade glances. She knows what I know. Let them alone. See what they can do.

First the wails and protests. Then the claims and rants. Finally the slaps and punches and scratches and pulling of hair. Bodies tumble onto the floor. Chairs overturn. Things that are thrown crash into the walls. The riot builds to a crescendo.

Angie and I lock eyes. This should do it.

I hear Mom first, at the top of the stairs. Stumbling in a stupor, with the smallest of her brood tucked like a football under her arm. She is wearing a long, silky Hawaiian-print summer nightgown with a zip-up front. Her hair is matted on one side, pushed toward her face, fuzzy and frayed around the edges like a shag she hasn't raked in days. Her face is blank.

I would have guessed Angry Mom would appear, frustrated, driven to tears. But no. It's not her. I can't read her puffy eyes as she thumps down the stairs, flat-footed and pained, clunking along like a piece of cartoon furniture. She comes to me and hands off Baby Joey without a word.

To Angie she says, "Feed the baby. Bottles are in the fridge." Her voice is flat, her body drained by the effort of coming down those stairs.

Angie and I trade worried looks.

This is a new mom, strange, apathetic. This is not even Dark Mom. She is blank, empty, spent, a breath exhaled for too long.

The hours pass slowly. By afternoon the heat brings out the smell of dirty diapers, spilt milk, and rotting fruit, the smell of all of us and her as well.

"Okay, everyone get in the Bronco." Mom is standing slumped in the living room, still in her nightgown.

"Where are we going?" I ask.

She doesn't answer but sets about herding kids. One by one she shoos us to the door.

A ride in the Bronco? Where will we go in our pyjamas and with our bed-heads in the middle of the afternoon? Where will she take Daniel and Brad with their dirty diapers and sticky fingers? Isn't she worried about Sunni, with her hair a nest of steel wool at the back of her head? What about me and Angie, unkempt, half-dressed, and greasy? She doesn't even have a diaper bag for Baby Joey. This is the mom who never wants us to cause a scene? We *are* a scene.

The Bronco is new, a nice ride with soft blue seats and four-wheel drive. It doesn't offer enough seat belts, but there is plenty of room for all of us to sit if we squish in or hold the little ones on our laps. We file into the Bronco, lifting each other through the high doors and up into the cab. Mom's quiet is eerie. She doesn't shush us as we snarl at each other about seats and who will be in the front. She doesn't care who sits where or who is poking whom. I take my seat behind her and watch her face in the rear-view mirror. Cold? Sad? I can't tell. A sense of urgency is in the Bronco—no, more inside my mind. I hear a voice calling to me from the back of my head. My Girl in the Back Brain. She knows more than I do about Mom today, she senses danger. *Is there danger?* She senses fear. *Is there fear?* Yes, I feel its first inkling.

As I watch Mom's face in the rear-view mirror I shrink a little inside my head and allow room for My Girl to move forward in case I need her. The door locks snap. Mom pulls the Bronco into reverse.

The sun is bright today. Long shadows lie across the road like dark silk trailing from the forest of wood and fern. If you look at just one spot, the dense wood of evergreen and birch blocks the view from the road. Only if you stare into the beyond and let the near edge blur to green as the trees slide by can you see deep into the forest. It is dark in there, too, and scary.

Mom turns down a narrow road that we seldom travel. I catch my breath at the view through the front window. The road winds on through a canopy of lush green brushed by a breeze, clouds dancing above the green. Some leaves are showing the first hint of change, tips of gold on a dressing of low-lying bushes. It's late August, with an early fall on the horizon, back to school, new friends, a new adventure just around the corner. I want things to be fresh. I want a bath. I want to feel clean again.

The rhythm of the tires slapping across tar lines on the asphalt road is a slow bass drum for the music of this drive. The bass strums through the floor of the Bronco while the shadows and light play a melody in my eyes. Shade and sun flicker like strobe lights. A quick blinding flash as the sun breaks through, then the strobe again through heavy leaves and branches, darkening for a moment inside a tunnel shot through the forest. Flickers and flashes. ·

I recognize this drive. Dad took us in the boat last week, four of us in orange life jackets, the engine gurgling, then roaring, the spray of the river cold on our faces, wet on our laps, soaking our feet. "It's a rough river this year, kiddos," he'd called from the back of the boat. His body turned to reach the motor's handle, steering the boat around the sandbars and jutting rocks, using the motor's gurgles and roars.

I love my speed-demon Dad, so daring, so happy, fighting the currents to avoid the sandbars. I love the rough river, no peace in it, the butterflies crashing into the walls of my stomach, the suspense with every oncoming obstacle. Would we make it? Would we crash?

"I'd hate to see this river high," Dad yelled. The boat turned us sideways and slammed us into a sandbar.

"Whoa, hang on, kids!" We screamed as we felt a shoosh of sand on the bottom of the boat, a sandbar eager to snatch the bottom of the boat right off. We cheered as Dad cleared it with a hearty prolonged roar. Finally we docked the boat and he lifted us out one by one. We were wet, excited, and cold. Going to the river in the Bronco was a happy time with Dad in the driver's seat and the boat hitched to the back.

This is different. This is a new, strange mom. And no boat.

I hear her voice, robotic, flat, but certain. "It's time."

Her tone terrifies me. *Time?*

Does she not hear the music of the ride? Is there not a single point of light for her among those flickers of light? How can she be so dark and cold?

Time for what?

I am afraid without knowing why. The little ones don't feel my feeling yet, and I am too afraid to stay there to tell them. Instead, I step back in my head to a safer place and leave everything to My Girl. She was right to be ready. She steps up and stands in my place. She questions and protests and keeps the memory so I can watch. "Time for what?" she asks. "Stop," she says. "I want to go home. Take us home, Mom, please, please, *please*."

In my memory, kept by My Girl, I see this moment like the shadows and light strobing across the road. I hear My Girl protest, beg, and cry. I see Mom's set mouth in the rear-view mirror. She's annoyed at My Girl, but she speaks to me. "Settle down, Autumn Dawn."

The time has come.

The Bronco is filled with the others but is an empty shell to me. Now only Mom and My Girl are here, as everyone else fades to the edges of my sight and hearing.

The Bronco slashes through the shadow tunnels, faster now as the bass drum of asphalt and tires picks up in pace, thrumming and throbbing. My ears pop as we descend into the valley.

The time has come.

The Bronco lurches at a break in the treeline. "No, Mom, please no, please, please, *please*." My Girl is screaming now, using my voice. I can see the river's muddy edge. I can see the roiling waters of the Peace River, wide and swift, the current dotted with sandbars that clog the river and black boulders that shred the surface, churning the water white with foam.

There's a moment of calm in the Bronco as Mom pulls past the break in the forest, past the boat launch, down the road, and out of sight of the enraged waters. The Bronco glides on the pavement, but Mom's jaw is still set, and her eyes are as blank as ever. Until a flash of determination pulls her face into a grimace. Her sudden U-turn amid the shadows brings back the screaming.

Nobody has said anything. But everybody knows now. *The time that has come is not a good time.*

The humming asphalt gives way to crunching gravel. Then a slosh against the water. The Bronco is moving down the launch, not backward the way Dad drives to set our boat in the water. We are going front-first. The slope is steep, and the view through the windshield is dizzying, nothing but water sweeping by: tiny, sucking whirlpools and deep, muscular ripples, sweeping by in a rush. From beneath the swirling surface come the sound and feel of gravel slipping, crunching, and grinding beneath the tires. Inside the Bronco the screaming builds.

Angie and Sunni and I have seen this river up close. We know what it can do. "No, Mommy, please no." My Girl screams for me. I am stuck behind My Girl, stuck with no place to look, no place where the rushing water does not rise up to engulf the Bronco as it creeps forward. I go far back into my brain, trying to shut out the shrieks. But I can still see flashes of detail.

Angie, holding baby Joey in the front seat, is screaming.

Sunni, her hands on the windows, is screaming and begging—she can see the water all around us now.

Daniel and Bradford are lost in the din, crying, but not certain why, our fear infecting them.

Baby Joey is oblivious to the danger but wailing anyhow.

And I, tucked away in the back of my brain, let My Girl cry out for me. My Girl grips the back of Mom's seat and bounces and howls. She stomps her feet and shakes Mom's seat. She begs and begs and begs as I slip deeper into the silence. Until the only sound I hear is the slap of the water on the Bronco. The rhythm and rocking, the throb of the foamy, cold water.

Mom's mouth in the rear-view mirror forms the words, "We'll all feel better soon." *The time has come.*

My Girl screams, *I don't want to die. I don't want to die. I DON'T WANT TO DIE.*

Until there are no more words amid the screams, and all that's left of screaming is a roar, a sound no longer in my ears but inside my head. Until . . .

The Bronco stops. The Peace River doesn't. It pulses darkly against the tires, rocking us inside, slapping up against the doors, nudging at the Bronco, licking, lapping, waiting, waiting.

Like a camera flash, Mom bursts. She melts over the steering wheel, wracked with sobs, slouched and broken. The tears come in waves, like the lapping of the river. She cries with a depth and an agony that I have never seen in her. My Girl and all the kids stop crying to watch her. My mom, tortured and lost and so desperate.

It's okay, says My Girl. *It's okay now. She won't hurt you. She doesn't really want to die either. It's okay.*

The Bronco backs away from the water's edge. It sits dripping for a long time. Until Mom drives away from the launch, still in tears, to take us for a ride not filled with terror. We drive for a long time. Until finally the last of the sobbing subsides and exhaustion sets in. I slump back in my seat and watch the shadows and hear the music of the drive again. Before My Girl settles back into her place, she tells me: *Now that Mom is crying and filled with emotion, everything will be okay again.* And it's true. That scary empty-eyed stare is gone. Her pain is better than her nothingness, this I now know.

I know that tonight there will be dinner and family prayer in the living room, pyjamas, and bedtime. I know we won't talk about the river. We won't talk about any of this. Mom will smile when Dad gets home, and we will sleep and put away this tortured memory. We will keep the hope that this memory won't ever come back to life.

Except it does come back, in my own life. Many years later, in a phone call to Dad.

"I'm really struggling with this pregnancy, Dad. I just can't get my head under control. It's so dark sometimes. I think it might kill me."

"Are you safe?" He knows these words of mine. He has heard them before from Mom, and they frighten him. "Autumn, I want you safe."

I shift the phone from one ear to the other as I roll over in bed.

"I'll be okay. I'll tell you, though, this baby has given me a new compassion for Mom. She must have been hurting so badly. She must have been so desperate that day."

"What day?"

"The day she drove us all down to the Peace River."

"What?"

"The day she told us all that it was time."

"*What* time? What are you talking about?"

I told him.

"What? Where was I?"

"I don't know, I think you must have been at work. It was at the end of summer, just before school started—after Joe was born . . ."

"Why didn't anyone tell me?"

How could you not have known? "Wow, Dad, I guess we just thought you knew. Kids always think that moms and dads know about stuff like that."

"If I'd have known, it wouldn't have happened."

He didn't know. It wouldn't have happened. Wow.

He didn't even believe it after I told him. He called Angie to confirm it.

7

When baby Joey was two months old, Dad turned twenty-eight. Mom was twenty-seven and a mother of six. Mom tried to make Dad happy, I know. As a surprise gift to him, she put up a wallpaper mural on the big wall in our living room. It was a nature scene with a crystal blue waterfall, shadowy trees, and a sunset over a forest of autumn colours. The browns and reds matched our calico brown and orange carpet—shag, of course—but none of the colours looked right against the paisley couch.

Even with the mural's mirage of open space, the Peace River house was too small for six children. Within a year our family moved fifteen minutes away, into the town of Grimshaw to live in a house tucked back on a quiet street. The house was dark brown with tan trim and it had an angular arch over the front section that made it look like an old-fashioned barn. There were groups of scantily blooming orange and yellow marigolds under the front window, and there was a doghouse at the side of the yard that smelled of wet animal dander and made me want to puke every time I passed by it. The lawn was as rough as any patch of prairie, and the yard was squat and narrow, opening onto a muddy alley and a poorly gravelled parking pad. The house was large, five levels stacked around short staircases. Two of the levels were basements, unfinished, with room to spare for visiting company.

Grimshaw. The sound of the name alone might have foreshadowed what was to come.

Life in Grimshaw brought some big changes for me. Mom grew tired of my hysterics when she tried to comb out my tangles. "Quit your whining or I'll take you in and have your hair chopped off." I didn't quit and finally she made good on her threat. The cut was a classic early-eighties style—shaved short at the back and flopped and teased and feathered at the front. My skinny body looked all the more skinny and my bony nose all the more prominent.

"And what can I get for you, little boy?" the lady at the ice cream counter asked.

"I'm a girl," I said.

"Oh," she said. "I really thought you were a boy."

"Everyone thinks I'm a boy."

"You should get your ears pierced or something."

My name didn't help. Dawn Stephan sounded like a boy. And my family called me Dawny when Donny and Marie Osmond were popular.

In grade three I saw a chance for a clean start. New school, new kids, new name. I decided to put my first name first. In class the teacher called the roll: "Don Steven . . . Don Steven? Raise your hand if you are here."

"My name is Autumn Stephan," I said, STEH-fun. And so, at school, I was. At home the struggle grew into tantrums. "My name is Autumn." The more I howled, the more my sisters called me Dawny.

One night, when Sunni and I were doing supper dishes, I found a newer, higher pitch, and Mom came flying into the kitchen to shut me up. She saw more than just a screaming match between two small girls. She grabbed me by the arm and hauled me up to her room.

"What is going on with you?"

"Sunni keeps calling me Dawny. I'm Autumn now. I'm not Dawny any more."

She finally heard me through the shrill of my tantrum. I could see it in her eyes. *At last.* "Why do you suddenly think you need to change your name?"

I couldn't tell her that I wanted to change my life, that I thought I was not worth the air I breathed. I couldn't tell her about hating school or hating home or hating my scrawny, sickly, wimpy body. I couldn't tell her that other girls looked like princesses, while I felt ugly and clumsy and worthless, that they could write in bubble letters and fancy curly handwriting on the blackboard while my writing looked like chicken scratches. I couldn't tell her that I had the biggest feet in the class. I couldn't tell her about the grinding need inside of me, the pain of simply being me. I couldn't talk about needing to be someone else. I could never say any of those things. So . . .

"The lady at the Super A thought I was a boy. I'm too skinny and everyone thinks I'm a boy."

My emotions broke from some place deep inside and rushed into my throat, choking me. There was so much more to say, but I'd never have her for long enough. There'd be another fight to settle downstairs. Or she'd just lose interest in me. "I even look like a boy."

"C'mon now, Autumn Dawn, don't screw up your face like that, it won't help you feel any better. Look at yourself." She touched my shoulder, turning me toward her bedroom mirror. "You look ugly when you cry like that." Her touch was kind enough, her tone soft. But . . .

I look ugly?

It isn't enough for me to say it? She has to repeat it?

Still. The next Saturday she took me down to the local jewellery store to pick out stud earrings. I had my ears pierced long before the mandated age of twelve. The sting of the piercing was sweet, an easy price to pay. After all the yelling and screaming I'd done, she'd heard me. Finally. That satisfied a need that I didn't know I had. Mom called me Autumn from then on. So my sisters had to call me Autumn. I was Autumn.

But my change in names and my new earrings were nothing compared to the changes in Mom. She had tried mothering and found it wanting. Her children, now nine, eight, six, four, three, and nearly one, had outgrown infancy and become independent souls. They were no longer snuffling, sniffling, sucking babies devoted to her and her alone. She had always set one child aside to bear another baby, each more needy than the last. But now home wasn't fulfilling enough.

Although we didn't need the income, she took a job at Croydon's Pizza as a cook and started her own woodworking company. She had always been creative, and now she poured an incredible amount of energy into her home business. She took over the lowest basement, building clocks on slices of log, rustic with a trim of jagged bark around the edge, delicate with yellow and cream rings decorated with decoupaged photos of family members or cut-outs from Norman Rockwell prints. She set up a booth in the mall to sell her crafts.

But still this did not fulfill the craving inside her.

She was absent, elusive, a shadowy figure who passed by now and then but never stayed put long enough to get to know me or the other kids as we continued to grow up. She was no longer at the door, waving and blowing kisses as we stepped out into the street on our way to school. She was no longer in the kitchen when we got home. Gone was the smell of freshly baked cookies after school. Gone was the comfort of an off-key melody lilting from the sink to the front door when we came in.

As the distance grew between Mom and the family, she shored up the boundaries and built herself a fortress with a midnight job. She began working at a group home for troubled teenagers. She had grown up in a house filled with foster children. She knew how tough it was to be noticed, let alone loved and needed. Maybe, as we her own children grew up, fighting among ourselves, fighting for our own identities, throwing tantrums to rename ourselves, we drove her from us. Maybe she found us too ungrateful for all she'd given us. Or maybe we just weren't needy enough any more.

The group home was full of abused teens, kids with wrecked lives, kids who needed protection from their parents and, in some cases, from themselves. If she needed the needy, she found them there in spades. And now that she worked all night, she slept all day.

"Mom, Mom? Can I go over to Julie-Anne's house to play?" I touch her bare arm, chilled above the covers.

She mumbles between sticky lips and gritted teeth.

"Can I go over to Julie-Anne's house to play? It's after school. We want to ride our bikes."

"Get out of here. Don't you come in here waking me up over dumb stuff. Get your can to the kitchen and make a snack for the boys. I don't want to hear you until I get up."

The boys are hungry and need to be entertained? Who has watched them all day while she slept? I make peanut butter crackers and a big mess and wait for someone else to come home. Eventually the house is full, and Dad puts a supper together. Mom is still not here with us. She wants what we can't give her. *But what?*

"I missed out, y'know." Mom is at the kitchen table, leaning on her elbow, resting her face on her hand. She is chatting with a woman who has come to board with us. Rebecca is tall and thin, and talented. She spends every night on the couch with a tiny metal crochet hook and fine, creamy cotton floss. I watch her fingers fly and marvel at the cloth she is making as loops and bumps counted carefully reveal a picture of Jesus at the Last Supper. She smiles a lot and tries to help around the house when she is there. Rebecca is in her early twenties; she is a member of our church and is staying with us as she works in a nearby town.

"I missed out on being a teenager. I had to work and survive, and I married so young. It's my turn to have some fun." Mom is close to tears, but her voice is quick and deliberate and determined.

Fun? She needs fun? At the time I heard her say it, having fun seemed almost reasonable to me because I was only eight and living for fun myself. Yet I felt the gentlest of nagging pangs. Mom wants to have fun without us? Why? Why not have fun *with* us?

8

Soon enough, Mom began spending more time with the teens than with us. When her shift was over, she met them after hours. Mom was not isolated on the acreage any more, and for the first time since she married at seventeen, she found herself the alpha female in a social group where every other member was at least twelve years younger.

"What the crap were you thinking?" Dad is in the kitchen with Mom and one of the group home girls. I am in bed. Mom has been gone for a few days straight; I've seen her only in passing. I am curious about where she has been.

"Oh lighten up, Stephan. It was just a little bit of fun. You should have seen me go, I'm a better climber than you could have guessed." There is laughter, like teenage giggles, but it is not funny to Dad.

"I don't know what you think you are doing, Deb, but I'm not going to be bailing you out for stupid stuff like this. You want to hang around with kids? Climbing the water tower? You could have gotten yourself killed."

I see Mom in my mind, hanging from her ankles, high above the town, like a child on the largest monkey bars ever built . . . and then the police drive up. The image makes me both smile and shiver. I fall asleep to the sound of mumbles and titters and grumbling from the kitchen.

Acting out teenage fantasy wasn't enough for Mom. She allowed several of the group home kids to move in with us. We doubled up bedrooms. New walls were slapped up in the open basement out of two-by-fours and drywall and screws.

Strangers filled the corners of our home, boys with guitars and girls with black eyeliner wearing jeans that mothers who have borne six babies don't stand a chance of struggling into.

"I'm too fat," I hear her tell Rebecca. "Hopelessly fat. I weighed in at the gym today at a hundred sixty." Mom is crying about it in the kitchen. Again. She cries a lot these days.

"Debbie, you've had six babies, and just look at you."

"No."

"Yes, you look great."

"No, I'm starting a new diet tomorrow, and I'm going to start doing those dance aerobics in the mornings again."

Diet. The diets when Mom eats only grapefruit or drinks only lemonade with cayenne pepper. Or eats only brown rice. Mom was never happy on a diet. But dance aerobics? I like the sound of that. And it means I can be with Mom.

We dance in the living room. The steps are fun, and the music makes me want to hoot with joy. We clap and turn, shake it, and hop to the silly tunes and the instructor on the tape. We step-tap-step-tap-step-tap-tap to the music, moving in a circle or a line until we are sweaty and desperate for a drink of water.

We laugh and sing along and stumble around the living room bumping into each other and twirling and shaking. Mom is so good. She loves dancing, and it is so great to be dancing with her even if I can't get the steps the way she does them. Step-cross-step-cross, shuffle left, toe-touch, shuffle right, clap and turn. I stop to watch her, to marvel at her agility and rhythm. I want to be a dancer just like Mom, in her powder blue shorts and sock feet.

"Are you staring at my crotch?" Mom stops dancing and covers her shorts with her open hands.

"No, Mom, I . . ."

"You filthy pig, get out of here." I turn to leave. Rebecca and the other girls are quiet as the red rises to my face.

"We don't stare at people's crotches, Autumn. That's perverted." She step-kicks at me as I run from the room. I wasn't staring at her. I didn't mean to see her crotch. I just wanted to be a dancer, and she is such a good dancer.

Later I tried to tell her. "Mom, I wasn't looking at your—"

"Hush, never mind."

"No, Mom, I—"

"Nope, drop it." Not letting me tell her I was not a pervert.

She spent more and more time out of the house. Her little time at home she spent in bed. She always looked so naturally beautiful back on the acreage, so insightful in her eyes, so loving in her soft mouth. Now she took to wearing her makeup hard, her black eyeliner and heavy mascara turning insight into anger. She painted her lips in skin tones and high gloss, going from soft to stony. I hardly knew her.

She cried a lot when she was alone—and she acted as if she were alone even if the six of us were home with her. She grew animated, even wild, when her new young friends would come around for coffee. Mom let them smoke in the yard and swear and laugh about things that we never talked about in our acreage home. The tension between Mom and Dad was thick. She was as rebellious and sarcastic as any of the teens from the group home. I was embarrassed for Dad.

"I'm not doing this any more, Deb. Do you hear me? You had better snap out of this crap or you are going to find yourself on the street." Dad is yelling in the bedroom. I cannot sleep through their skirmishes.

"Shut up, stupid, it's not crap and I'm taking my turn now. I don't need you acting like you're my father. These kids are my friends, and they need me. You aren't kicking anybody out of this house." Mom is angrier than I have ever heard her.

"This isn't a house, this is hell, and you've got a bunch of little kids who need their mother, not some crazy teenage freak."

"Oh, and you are just so perfect, Tony. You never do anything wrong, right?"

The screaming turns to whispers: heated, ugly, shrouded words behind the bedroom door. I am jolted by the sound of some shattered glass. I duck to hide under my covers.

Our world began to split into two camps. On one side were Dad and the kids. On the other were Mom and her friends. I missed being called to dinners of pasta and corn. I missed the chaos, the chatter of everybody butting in to tell their story of the day and elbowing to get at the butter first so they could slather it over the corn. I missed my dad's easy smile. Part of him never came to the table when she was gone. And I missed my mom.

Mom did come home at last. She was so sick that she had to quit most of her hobbies and all of her work. She came home, but not in the way I'd dreamed.

The teens from the group home stayed with us still. They brought their troubled lives with them, their hard rock, their drugs, their drinking, their in-your-face nakedness with their bedroom doors wide open. They brought their resentments, rages, turmoil, and terror. They couldn't have been all bad, surely. But they were teens, with their revved emotions and their rampant hormones. And they came from bad pasts, all victims of abuse and neglect, all schooled in violence. Surely there were good days while they stayed there at the house with us. But all I can remember is the terror.

"What do you think you're doing coming into this house stoned?" I wake to the sound of Mom screaming. I struggle to get off my sagging foam mattress, which hangs deep in the loose springs of the metal cot. The room is dark and hot, illuminated only by the bright light streaming under my new unpainted door. I teeter on the edge of the foam and wait to listen for more. Sunni is still in her bed across the room. I can see that her eyes are open wide.

"What are you doing up? Just go to bed, Mother dear." It is the voice of the girl Mom favoured above all the others.

"You should have been in hours ago."

I hear the girl shuffling and stumbling in the kitchen. "Look at you," Mom yells. "You're knock-down drunk, stoned out of your stinking mind." Heavy objects hit the floor. *Thud, thud.* "I told you if you ever came back this way again, you'd be out. Do you hear me? You are out." Mom has gone from being a cool friend and a bit of an enabler to being a motherly figure and disciplinarian. The switch is not going over well.

Now there are strings of curse words. Words I don't know, mingled with the hair-raising sound of screeching furniture.

"I'm not going anywhere, Mother dear." The girl is breathy, and Mom is screaming now in a voice that I have never heard.

Sunni leaps from her bed and we huddle together behind the bedroom door—squatting low to the ground, holding the door and each other for balance.

"Should we go help Mom?" I ask in a whisper.

"No, we better wait here," Sunni says. She is shaking and grinding her teeth.

Smashing.

Swearing.

Screaming and thumping.

Dad's tired voice. "Hello, officer, we need you here immediately. My wife's been attacked by one of our boarders."

I open the door to run to Mom, but the girl is still in the house. She sees me and screeches, "Oh, stop crying, you dumb little bitch." Then she turns her rage back on Mom: "Deb, you're raising a bunch of bloody babies in this house."

I can't stop howling, but I run behind my door again as she lunges toward me. "You want me to come in there and give you something to cry about, you stupid little bitch?"

I slam my door, and Sunni and I hold it shut, pressing against it with all our little-girl weight. She doesn't even try to come in.

Dad yells to us, "Just stay in there, girls. Wait for the police."

By now Sunni and I are hysterical. We can hear crying from the kids in the other rooms as well. The ranting and screaming and smashing don't end. We hear our names amid the swearing and thrashing about. We hear Mom crying and begging the girl to stop. We hear Dad pummelling the girl, trying desperately to protect Mom from the monster she has invited into our lives. We hear the police enter, new voices taking charge of the situation. Finally, blessedly, we hear the silence.

They take her away. Dad comes in to tuck all of us back into bed. "It's over," he says. "Go to sleep. It's okay now."

Next day a battered Mom said the girl would never be back. She was done with trying to help people who didn't want help. It was all I could do not to jump for joy.

The joy was silent and short-lived because Mom changed her mind—
even before the bruises healed—and took the girl back. She said everyone needs a home and a family, even girls who have big problems.

9

Our family packed up and moved to the far northern city of Fort McMurray, which brought new schools, new work for Dad, and a new home—much smaller than the Grimshaw barn. This boxy split-level covered in aluminum siding had no personality. It was the same as every other house on the block, with its flat face, large front window pane to the right, two smaller windows to the left, and a screen door between. Three basement windows looked out to the front, their view guarded by overgrown bushes and a few scrawny flowers in a narrow, unkempt garden space. The only difference among the houses was the colour. Ours was cream, trimmed in brown.

Broken blocks of cement formed a sorry sidewalk that led to the rutted asphalt road. I could look across the road toward a new northern vista beyond, this one with more trees than in Grimshaw, this one promising eternal peace cloaked in green. I could go there to get away, walking among the tall swaying birches and thick stolid evergreens crowding each other, the birches spreading out at the top to steal the light, the evergreens spreading out below to get the better footing. The trees guarded my path through the damp undergrowth. My path. A path, deep and shady, at times dark. I would cut through the air, soupy with gnats and mosquitoes, and try not to inhale them with the dank smell of rotting leaves and fresh baby ferns.

Beyond the trees the land rolled into a deep valley, sopping wet with river and marsh. My path ended at a cliff overlooking a sea of green below, a sea speckled with housetops and parted at its deepest by a winding ribbon of crystal blue, the Athabasca River.

My spot. My one comfort, in the open where the wind could find me and dust away the sadness and lighten my heavy heart. Where the breeze could keep the legions of frenetic, spindly mosquitoes beyond arm's length. Here I was one with the trees, one with the soil and the ferns and the moss, one with the wind. Here at least, in this singular spot on earth, life was good. I felt like a part of the greater creation. I went there often for renewal I could not find at home or in the new town.

In Fort McMurray there was a chance to start over—to make new friends and new reputations for ourselves. It worked for Mom, but she wouldn't let it work for me.

"Okay, so Autumn is a bit of a scatterbrain," she said to a woman from our new church. "She's really emotional, y'know? Kids in Grimshaw called her Old Yeller." She snickered and covered her mouth.

The woman had come calling, bringing a meal for the newcomers. My introduction.

"She's lazy and really has a tough time making friends. I get so frustrated with her. I'll give her a project to work on and she gets halfway and then never finishes it. She's got no attention span and no desire to stick to anything."

Later I imagine how I might have introduced her to the same woman. *This is Debbie. She's a bit confused. Okay, so sometimes she thinks she's a mother and sometimes she thinks she's a sixteen-year-old. She's a bit mean sometimes. Oh, but she can be nice, too. Trouble is, you never quite know until she either kisses you on the cheek or smacks you in the mouth. Are you sure you want to be her friend? She can be a handful. Especially when she turns on you. Which she will do, eh? Well, hey, you can be her friend if you like. I mean, it's a free country. Okay, so don't ever say I didn't warn you.*

Of course, I could never have done that to her. Nine-year-olds can only think of rants like that in bed, at night. Never on the spot, never when it counts. And that's a good thing because had I ever said anything like it, she would have killed me.

I wanted to be done with Grimshaw. I wanted it to be my past. Instead, she made it the foundation for what I would become. Had she thought of me in that way all along? How did I miss it? How did she even notice what I was like in Grimshaw, where she was so engrossed in her turn at

having fun that she had no time for her family? *That's what I was to her?*
Old Yeller? Lazy? Friendless? Shiftless? That's all?

How would I ever get those words out of my head?

"Why are you crying, Autumn?"

My school teacher is leaning over my desk, sheltering my face from
the other kids in the room. I can't get my feelings under control. I want
to run out of the room but I'm not allowed to do that. She touches
my shoulder, and I feel a charge of comfort and strength run through
me. She's worried about me. She cares. Her concern is all I need to
stop the tears.

"I can't do this math." I come up with the most benign reason I can
think of for crying.

"Well, maybe your school in the Peace Country didn't keep the same
schedule. Let's see if we can do some review pages first." She flips
through my book to a section of grade three review. I plough through it
in no time because I want to impress her, because I want to show her I
am not lazy, not shiftless. She is left baffled, searching my swollen eyes
for an answer I cannot give her.

My grade four school teacher was the first of many to notice that I
had a problem: inconsistency, moodiness, quick tears, and quick rage. It
was the ebb and flow of my emotional tides, the swings in everything
Autumn. There were days when I did no work at all. Then there were
days when I did so much she thought I must be cheating.

"Autumn, did you write this?" My teacher has my report in hand,
titled "All About the Brain," as she hovers at my desk.

"Yes."

"Can I see you at the back, please?"

She pulls a chair up to the back table and sits down with a pile of
books.

"Do you know what plagiarism is?"

"No."

"It's copying someone else's work from a book and calling it your own.
It's not okay to do that. It's cheating." She shoves the pile of books at me.
"Could you please show me which book your report came from?"

"I used lots of books, but I didn't copy them. I just used the books for the learning part." I'm in trouble, the tears are welling up, and my face is getting red.

"Autumn, this is not grade four work."

"Why?"

"It's just not. Tell me where you copied it from."

"I didn't, it came from my head. I didn't copy it. I didn't." I am crying. My fists are angry and tight and I am escalating into a fit. The kind of tantrum that forces Angela to stop bugging me before Mom comes in and smacks her for making me scream and waking up the house. The kind of fit reserved for self-preservation, attention-grabbing, or forcing a bigger person to back down. The kind of fit that makes Mom call me Old Yeller.

"Shh, okay, Autumn, it's okay. You aren't in trouble, I'm not mad. I just wanted to know where your report came from."

I didn't cheat. I didn't cheat. I cry into my arms folded on the table. And she doesn't believe me. And now she knows I am odd, besides.

My teacher arranged for me to be tested by the school psychologist. When the tests came back, everyone was shocked, including me. The woman who tested me with pictures and puzzles and math and paragraphs of writing and reading came to get me from class. I liked her. She smelled good and she was soft-spoken and smiley. "Autumn, please come to the library."

I join her on the little chairs by the kindergarten reading section.

"We looked at your test results, and I wanted to tell you about them before we tell your parents."

"Okay." The red is rising in my neck. *My parents. I'm in trouble.*

"You see on this paper? These are the numbers for your work. If there were one hundred children being tested, you did better than ninety-eight of them. And in one area, you did better than most teenagers would do, even adults. Except for math, where you do as well as most of your classmates, and that's okay, because you can be average and be perfectly happy with that."

"What's average?"

"Just like everyone else."

"Oh." I want to be like that. Just like everyone else.

"There's just one thing I wanted to talk to you about." I sit up straighter. "On the timed reading portion of the test you got only half of it done. But the part you finished was one hundred percent correct. You understand very well, but I think you were just being too careful and so you worked slowly. It's okay for you to read faster. If you work on that, you will be brilliant."

Brilliant? She thinks I might be brilliant? Brilliant like a star? I can't tell her the truth. I can't tell her that I was slow because the words wandered on the page and my eyes couldn't stay on the right line. I can't admit I have to read the same line, tracing it with my finger, over and over until the letters lift from the page and sink into my mind. I want to tell her: I know the words and they are beautiful and I love reading. If only it didn't take such a long time for the words to go from the page to my brain.

But I don't tell her, and she keeps talking about the puzzles and my quick problem solving and my excellent story and the way the story gave her chills because it wasn't grade four work. She enrolls me in "Gifted and Talented Extracurricular Studies."

I feel like a fraud. I should have told her how hard it was for me to read. But I was afraid that if I did, she would take it all back. You have to trace each line over and over? Oh, well. Maybe not so brilliant, not so talented. Back to the dunces with you then.

I don't tell her or anybody. Even so, I am excited to bring the letter home to Mom. I need to stand out in her eyes. Forget about gifted and talented studies. If I could be important to Mom, if I could give her a reason to be proud of me and to have something good to say about me. Just one good thing. *Please?*

I stand beaming in the doorway, clutching the letter. *Be proud of me.*

"Let's see." She stands with her dish towel over her shoulder, reading the crumpled letter. I watch a smile ease across her face. She traces down the page, running her index finger over the numbers. The closer she gets to the bottom, the wider her smile gets. I take it to mean she is proud. Barefoot and tired, and proud of me. At last. *Thank you, thank you, thank you.*

"This is good, Autumn, but I don't want it going to your head, okay? So don't go boasting about it or you won't get any friends."

"Okay, Mom."

"Okay, Genius. Come on in here and set the table."

I cringe. *Genius?*

Better than Loud Mouth or Scrawny. Or Scatterbrain. But . . .

"Do you think I really am a genius, Mom?"

"I'm not telling you. If I did, you'd get too snotty."

Well, it is an answer. She does believe what the letter says. But if she tells me what she thinks, I'll get snotty. Lazy. Friendless. Shiftless. Old Yeller. Now she adds Snotty. And Genius. And not a regular genius, either. Snotty Genius.

10

Mom wasn't always vicious. She was often gentle, motherly, feminine, and kind, especially with Dad around. She was faithful and loving to him. To us, she was one of the television moms on the classic shows like *Leave It to Beaver*, the kind of wife who waved in the front window when Dad drove off to work, the kind of wife who called him to say, "Hello, I love you," in the middle of the workday. There was a lot of music in our home. There was still laughter between them, hand-holding across the aisle of the van between the bucket seats. Kisses in the kitchen. The smell of lobster tails and garlic butter wafting from the dining room at midnight.

Mom's love for Dad was the one sure thing in my life. They were a team. She wanted to be his partner in every way. When times got tough and Dad started his property management business, she dug in and carried her share of the burdens. She did the books for Dad's business. She said that they were going to work together from now on. I liked the sound of that word, *together*. But soon there was family business of another kind to attend to. Mom was pregnant. Again. And she was sick and so tired.

The babies were usually gifts for Mom. Little things she loved to wrap and unwrap, cuddle and sniff and kiss and rock to sleep. This time, though, Mom's baby was a gift for me, too, because it brought Shawna into my life. Shawna, my dearest friend.

We started out hating each other. Her dad was a teacher in the public school, and so she thought she ran the place. My great introduction to Shawna? Cola in my milk. In Mom's world cola was poison; in Mom's world it was a propellant to hellfire. And I drank it, all because of Shawna. I faked nausea, put on a show for the lunchroom, spitting and spilling and trying to vomit on my cafeteria tray. Shawna laughed, and the girls with her snickered and then roared when I started crying. I didn't care, really. Anything to be sure that God knew it wasn't my choice to drink cola.

Shawna had a weakness, and I did, too. I needed a friend, and she needed babies. She was the youngest in her family, and she was looking for a place to go and little people to care for. One day we were forced to talk to each other while waiting for rides home from school. Her dad was taking way too long to leave the school, and my mom was trying to get there but got tied up with the little kids. I was stuck with Shawna in the front entrance between the big glass doors. We leaned our butts against the boot racks and stared at the roof and the ceiling and kicked at the mud rugs. When we had finished ignoring each other and were sure there was no one else around, we abandoned our disdain and chatted the way all ten-year-old girls do.

"My mom's having a baby."

"Really, can I come over?"

It was that simple, and Mom loved Shawna instantly. So having her over became the right thing to do.

Baby David was born chubby and doughy and round. His blond head was too big for his body, so we called him Tady, which is the nice way of saying potato head. Shawna came to play with Tady and me every day after school and often on weekends. We had sleepovers, and Mom let us move the big blue couch into my room so Shawna would have a place to sleep. We took care of Tady and pretended we were mommies.

Mom did okay for a while after Tady was born, but the broken sleep soon caught up with her. We were back to her silky zip-up pyjamas and puffy eyes and self-exile in her room. I didn't think much about it any more. I thought stay-at-home moms just didn't get dressed. I was going to be a working mom so I could wear real clothes and perfume and high heels when I grew up. That's what I thought.

Summer came, and it was a relief to Mom. During school months she had to get out of bed and scan the lot of us for signs of illness. Angie, are you fevered? No. Autumn, how's your skin today? Do you have sore skin? Yes? Oh, well, you had better stay home from school.

Staying home sick didn't mean resting, it meant running back and forth from Mom's bedroom to the kitchen, the bathroom, the laundry pile. It meant running the vacuum, the dishwasher, the laundry machines. But now that summer was here, Mom could call on anyone, any time. She stayed in bed all day. She never dressed.

Tady is nine months old, ready to fly the nest. "Mom, can me and Shawna take Tady downtown?"

Mom rolls over and peers through one fluttering eyelid.

"What?"

"Can we take Tady downtown, on the transit bus? We want to go to the mall. I have money from my allowance."

"Mmmm. Sure. Okay."

"Good, I'll bring a bottle for him, okay, Mom?"

"Mmmmhmmm. Okay."

II

The hallway from my grade five class leads to an exit on the side of the school. I am more than able to walk home alone. If I run into Sunni or Angela I will walk with them, but they have their own friends, and we make our own way after school is out.

I am glad school is over. I am glad to be going home. I don't like it here. I miss my grade four teacher and the principal from the public school. But Mom says the Catholic schools are better, and even though we are not Catholic, they teach good values. So I have had to leave my only friend, Shawna, and move to the Catholic school across the parking lot.

I have started all over again. A different gifted class, a different regular class. No friends. Nothing to lean on but my hope of graduating one day and leaving school behind.

I slam out the side door and step into a group of girls from my class. Uh-oh. There are some older girls, too, from Angie's grade. They are taller and wider than I am, and my heart flips over in my chest. I know these girls. They caught me on the playground just last week.

Kelly is the ringleader. She boasts about doing drugs and using Visine to clear her eyes before class. She's tough. I'm not. "There's Autumn. Oooh, she's so smart. Careful, don't touch her, you might get the cooties."

Another girl grabs my blouse. She pushes me into Kelly. They call me names. The smarty-farty. The ugly, stinky fleabag. They toss me back and forth and into the brick wall. My book hits the ground, open-faced. I get scrapes from the wall and scratches from fingernails.

"Oh, it's Mr. Vincent," one girl calls out, and the group disbands, leaving me against the wall.

"Mom! Mom! Mom!" My scream is shrill, piercing my own eardrums as I storm through the door. "Kelly and her team beat me up again! They pushed me and they said I was nerdy and they pushed me against the wall and they said I was stinky and they pushed me and they said I was ugly!" I jump up and down, shaking and screaming at the top of my lungs.

"You settle down right now, Autumn Dawn. Right now—I mean it." I don't stop, so she shoves me onto the back deck. The deck is raised, a second floor entry. It looks over the neighbours' fences, exposed to all the kitchen windows. "You can come in when you are ready to act normal." She shuts the door behind her, shuts me and my racket out of the house.

I keep screaming. My voice echoes off the houses and fences. Everyone can hear me. I don't care. Mom will just have to pay for pushing me out here instead of holding me close. She doesn't come. So I let loose. I scream every ugly word short of swear words. A few choice curses would bring her. But she would not hold me then. She'd drag me in by the hair and give me a good beating for my dirty mouth.

I grip my fists until my nails cut into the palms of my hands. I stomp and howl until the howling turns to moaning and the stomping turns to shuffling. Until I am spent.

It's over. She does not come. I stand on the deck in a sweat. The breeze flops my limp hair onto my face. I look down at my scrawny body. I am dressed in a frilly white blouse and a pair of stretchy pants and running shoes. I am not cool. I am not pretty. They are right about me, all of them. I am a freak. I am shiftless, lazy, and snotty. *I hate you,* I say to myself, going on an internal rant. *I hate you, I hate you, I hate you.*

I don't want to live any more.

So I begin plotting ways to die. There is the cliff at the end of my favourite path in the woods. They call it Suicide Hill. I imagine soaring through the air, a free fall to the rocks and the water below. I like the idea of flying. Very dramatic. Killing myself on Suicide Hill. It has a nice ring to it. Except. *Where's Autumn? Anybody seen Autumn these last ten years?*

They may never find me. The animals will eat my flesh. That's no good. Death is no good if nobody knows where I went or if nobody can identify the gnawed bones.

In the tub. I can do that. Slip my face below the bubbles. If I just take one deep breath of water, it might work. Mom will knock on the door at first. Then she will bang hard. The boys will dance outside the door and whine. *Hurry up, Autu-u-u-umn. We have to pee-e-e-e.* She will get angry and yell at me. And, being dead, I will not answer. They will use a hairpin to open the lock, and they'll come in and find me, floating pale and naked in the water. They will think it was a terrible accident. Except I don't want them to think it was an accident. *Poor girl slipped and fell on the soap. Just like in the cartoons.*

Then they won't know how desperate I was. They will just think it was a terrible, sad accident. That's no good. They have to know I meant it.

A fall in the road? In front of traffic? Not bad. They will find me bloody and gory and broken, and that's better than naked and shrivelled and soapy. But that's not good either. They might think I'm not smart. They might say I was stupid to be walking so close to moving traffic. *She tripped in front of a garbage truck? Maybe she wasn't so gifted after all.*

Dying. Not as easy as I thought, once I think about it.

I must have standards, criteria. If I am to die well, my death has to meet all of my criteria. I want out, but they need to know it and see it and feel it. Know it, see it, and feel it with guilt and pain and grief, terrible grief. They will have to miss me. Otherwise, dying is not worth the effort.

Mom will have to run to my body and know it was no accident. She must fall on her knees and beg forgiveness and howl as I did on the deck, following a script: *Poor Autumn. Poor, poor Autumn. She was so smart and good, hey, and I loved her and I wish I had told her and I wish I could take it back and hold her when she was sad instead of embarrassing her. Come back, Autumn, please, please, please. I need my little girl. I need you. I love you and not just because you are my child, hey, but because you are worth loving. Oh, poor Autumn. Poor, poor Autumn.*

A very pretty picture, that. But how to arrange it?

One day I walked into the kitchen to find Mom cutting up a raw chicken. I was fascinated by how easily the flesh was pierced with the knife. When the joints were approached properly, they just separated and the limbs fell away.

"Oh, poor chicken," I whispered under my breath.

"What did you just say?" asked Mom.

"Just 'poor chicken.' " I'd blown it now.

"Get out of here. I don't need you feeling sorry for the chicken when I have to stand here and cut it up."

Later that night, when Mom was tucking the boys in bed, I went into the kitchen alone. I got out the butcher knife and admired the curve of the blade. It was clean and cold, and the handle was black and easy to grip. I ran my hand over my T-shirt to find the place where the knife could enter without being slowed down by bone. I could feel every rib and every space between.

"Scrawny Dawny," I said so I could hear the sound of it. So disgusting. Destined to be a failure besides. Not just a lazy, snotty, shiftless, friendless Old Yeller. Other things, too. I spoke the names aloud: "Liar, Loud-mouth, Ugly, Dramatic, Sickly, Selfish, Hypochondriac, Cocky, Annoying. All-Round Pain in the Neck." All by the age of eleven. I held the knife to my chest and fantasized about how it could pierce a spot between my ribs. Just like a chicken joint. If I just fell forward on the blade—

You forgot Embarrassment. My Girl in the Back Brain. I stopped leaning and dropped my arm, letting the knife swing at my side. It was true. I forgot that I was an embarrassment, too. And being an embarrassment could be the worst sin of all. If I failed, they'd find me in a puddle of blood in the kitchen but still alive, and they would have to go to hospital and call Social Services. And I would be an embarrassment to the family. Not just a greasy, unkempt, tired little girl, but an embarrassment. No greater sin than that.

I put suicide aside until I could be sure I'd be good at it. Until then, I could hope. I could pray. Maybe God would take me. With luck, I would simply cease to exist. No Autumn. Just a memory.

When I was thirteen, I kept a journal. Each page was a print of blue sky and puffy clouds. There were quotations on the bottom of each page about dreaming big dreams, making dreams a reality. When I wasn't dreaming about suicide, I wanted to do big things, good big things. I told my journal I'd help people, teach people, build a house where hungry people could go and be fed and healed. I would be wealthy but not proud, and other people would be blessed because I was sharing.

I wrote about loving God and wanting to be helpful to Him. I wrote when I was happy or feeling poetic. When I was angry, I didn't write. I knew there were some things that should never be said in writing— some things that should never be read out loud.

I loved writing. The feeling of the pen on the paper. The feeling of the words spilling from my mind onto the page. When I read them later, it felt as if they were someone else's words I was seeing for the first time.

"Hey, Autumn, come in here." Mom is in her bedroom. She pats the flowery bedspread.

Wary, I climb up and sit by her.

"I saw a bit of your blue cloud dream journal pages. I didn't mean to snoop, but I was in your room, and the pages were loose and falling out, so I picked them up."

"Oh?" I'm suddenly glad I censor my writing.

"Anyway, I saw the part you wrote about you believing in God 'just because' and I thought we should have a talk."

Am I in trouble? In trouble with God? Will she add Heathen to my list of names?

"Mom—"

"It's okay, Autumn."

"All I meant was that I knew He cared and I couldn't explain why."

"I'm not mad. I just need to tell you about this. I need to tell you about a dream I had when I was pregnant with you. I think it is the reason you have such a strong personality and an automatic faith in God when others might struggle with it."

She had a dream? About me? I tip over onto my stomach. Mom does the same so we are lying beside each other like sisters, even friends. I stroke the flowers and pick the lint on the comforter as I listen to her open up her heart.

"When I was little, there was a lot of scary stuff happening in my home. My dad travelled and sold pots and pans, and my mom was stressed out and was really mean to my sisters and me."

I stop picking lint. *Your mom was mean to you, too?*

"What did she do?" *How much was she like you?*

"Well, it's not important." Her face is hard, her lips pursed. "All you need to know is that I was little and hurt and I wanted to die."

Oh! So did I, Mom. I wanted to die, too. "Mom—" *I even thought about throwing myself in front of a—*

"Hush."

—garbage truck.

"So, when I was a little girl . . ." She chokes on the words. "I heard in Sunday school . . ." She bites her upper lip. "That Jesus would come again."

Me, too, Mom. I prayed—

"I always prayed that . . . He would come and take me away from my mom . . ."

I didn't want to exist.

"And protect me from her . . ."

I'm sorry I said I hate you.

"And from the ugly world . . . "

Don't stop. Not now. Please keep talking.

"I had a dream when I was a little girl. Over and over again, I had that dream. That Jesus was coming, and everyone in the neighbourhood was running out of their houses to see Him."

She begins to get excited. She is still having that dream. Right now, in her eyes, I can see it.

"I could hear the sounds in the streets. All the excited children laughing and running to get to Him. But when I would run to the door, my mother would grab me and hold me so I couldn't go. She would just hold me. In the dark house. While all of the other children got away. I couldn't get past her."

Now the dream has become a nightmare in her eyes. She's seeing it in real time.

"I would wake up, after the dream, crying and praying that He would come to find me."

There are no tears in her eyes, just the nightmare. Her face is hard. All she wants is to get away. I know this feeling. It is my life. *She has lived my life before I lived it myself?* I lie in silence, not looking, not moving, not daring to breathe.

"So, after your dad and I got married, we moved away. It took me a while to realize that I was free. I had a lot of sadness about my mom and my dad. It took some time to feel like I was okay. Then, when I was nineteen, I was pregnant with you. And I had the dream again. It was exactly the same. The same dream as when I was a kid. It started out with me in the living room. Hearing the sounds in the street. And knowing that Jesus was coming. I wanted to go out. I ran to the door. I reached the door frame just as my mom grabbed my arm. But this time I slipped away from her. I tore out into the sunlight. I ran and ran and ran until I saw Jesus. I felt my feet leave the ground. He was standing above the ground on a cloud or something. I looked at his face and I felt the most intense feeling of love that I had ever known. My whole body was filled with light and love. I fell onto my knees and cried, and my tears dropped onto his bare feet. I went to wipe them off with my fingers. When I touched the top of his foot—the nail mark, in his flesh—my fingertips burned." She holds out her hand and brushes over the tips of her index, middle, and ring fingers with the soft pad of her thumb, feeling the memory of the burning even now.

She begins crying. The tears pool in her eyes, and she blinks them down onto her face. She can barely string her words into sentences.

"You were there. With me. You were. Inside me. When I met Him. I think that's why. You know Him. So well. That's why. Believing. In Him comes. So easily to you."

Her lips are pursed no longer. They are soft and wet, vulnerable, bitten.

"This was so. Real to me. So sacred. When I thought about it. My fingers. Burned. Even months later. They still burned. I know He lives, Autumn. I know He loves us. I know He will come again, and I want you to be ready when He comes."

I am filled. I love my mother. And I know that God loves her, too, and me; God loves me, and this is surely the feeling they told me about. The feeling of the Spirit. The warm feeling in my heart, the calm feeling in my mind that tells me what is true. *Thank you, God, for not letting me fall off the cliff or into traffic or onto that knife.*

"I just needed you to know that, Autumn."

"Thanks, Mom. I needed to know it, too. Thanks."

She takes a deep breath and wipes her face roughly. "Okay, so. We have stuff to do. You get the kitchen cleaned up." She turns her head and hollers, "Angela, are you out there? Did the bathroom get done?"

The moment is over. No more sisters. I slide off the bed and walk out on the miracle that just happened. Two miracles, really. One, she loves me; and two, she wants me to know it.

13

Shawna and I stayed friends, although we went to different schools. She just had to stay my friend. She loved babies, and Mom didn't let her down. After Tady was out of diapers, Mom had Jeremy. She called him Dustin for the first few days, but it didn't suit him, so she paid the money and sent in the papers to change his name to Jeremy. Shawna and I had a new toy. Jer Bear, the sweetest little boy we knew, with bright eyes and a laugh that filled the whole house when we pulled up his shirt and blew on his belly. Oh, the games we would play, tossing him in the air and kissing his belly and letting him chew on our knuckles. Jer Bear, the teddy bear, another gift from God.

Then Mom did it again. A sister. The smallest baby I had ever seen. She was born on Christmas Eve. Mom wanted to call her Celestial Starr. Dad said no way, and they argued the whole Christmas dinner and settled on Celeste. On her blessing day, she was still too small for clothes, so Mom dressed her in Sunni's Cabbage Patch Kid christening dress. A white lacy outfit with a cheap Velcro closure. Jeremy couldn't pronounce Celeste, so he called her CC. The name stuck.

We didn't get to hold CC often because she would get cold. Mom held her, wrapped in pink lace and soft flannel. She checked her temperature often. Mom's little dolly, her little baby girl to finish up a five-in-a-row streak of boys.

When CC turned one month old, I turned fifteen and became newly aware, seeing my mother in a new light. Normal, not normal—the terms simply do not cover the swings between Mom's terrifying rages and her happy, peppy highs.

"Hey, get in here and do the dishes. RIGHT NOW."

She never asks any more. She just yells. We could live with the yelling, I suppose, and the name-calling. But she's violent, too. We jump at the first demand or suffer a kick or a smack. She is tired and worn out, and I think she is lonely. Dad's service as volunteer clergyman in the church takes him away from us for long periods. He deals in properties, too, and business is at an all-time high. He flies his own private plane from city to city to manage government buildings and residential apartments. He is youthful and energetic and busier than ever. Mom flips between two moods. Not so much sadness now. But angry most days. Excited, bubbly, and musical the rest of the time.

Today I hear her yelling at the kids when I come up the front steps after school. "Clean up this damned mess. I've had it. Who left this book bag in the front entrance? Who?"

I wait. I stand outside praying she won't open the door and find me here standing stiffly. The yelling fades to another part of the house. *Whew*.

I slip in and take a spot at the table. My Girl coaches me. *Get productive. Show how hard you can work. Get the look. Get busy, girl. Homework.*

"Autumn, is that you?" All I did was open my book bag.

"Yes? I'm doing my—"

"Look what I brought home today." She stands in the hall. She has a shopping bag under her arm. All her clothes are new. This is Happy, Skippy, Spendy Mom.

"Wow, you went shopping." I am wary, very wary.

"Oh yeah, I got a couple new dresses and these pants and two tops and some hair pretties. Do you like?" She spins around like a model on a runway. She points her toe and lifts her pant leg to expose a sparkly silk stocking with embroidered flowers on it. Then she bows her head to show me the brass clip adorned with plastic rhinestones.

"Nice, Mom, that looks great." When she's dark and dangerous and on the prowl, I've learned to be submissive. When she's been spending money and is fake and breathy and giddy, I am even more careful. It means a quick temper. It means a fast, hot rage. At times like this, I humour her. Smile. Be pleased with her. Above all, I don't give her any offence to remember when she flips to the dark side. Because she will remember.

"Oh, so just a minute and I'll show you what else I got." She skips down the hallway and disappears into her bedroom.

I go back to my textbook, curious about the shopping but eager to look busy. She comes back holding a hanger. At first glance it's one of those flimsy plastic bags caught on a branch outside the window. But no, the hanger is draped with a limp white spandex dress. The dress looks small enough for a child, shorter than anything I would dare bring home. It's like a dance costume without the tulle skirt. Just a tube with puffy long sleeves. The forearms are tighter tubes covered in silver sequins. The neckline is high and fitted and sparkling with sequins as well. Definitely a dance costume. *Surely, she's not going to wear that thing.*

"Oh, it's beautiful. I—" I catch the look in her eye. Oh.

I cover my mouth so my braces don't show. I'm shocked. I have a school dance to go to tonight. "Oh, Mom." *Surely you don't expect me to—*

"I just saw it and thought, now that would be perfect for Autumn with her tight little bum and perky little body. Okay, so size six, right?"

I nod. *Surely not.*

"I just couldn't help it, I could just imagine you in it at the dance. So I got it." A big, happy, skippy, spendy Debbie smile. "For you."

She hooks the hanger on the knob of the china cabinet and hippety-hops past me into the kitchen. "Don't try it on yet, wait until after supper."

She shopped for me? She brought home nothing for the other kids? She said nice things about my figure? I don't know—maybe it really will look good on me. Maybe I am as perky as she says?

I'd like to see for myself, but I'm not about to push my luck and ask to try it on now. I'll do it her way. The dress hangs there for all to admire during supper. After the last plate is cleared, I snatch it off the knob and tear down the stairs to get ready for the dance.

The dress is skin-tight and sheer enough to show every snap and hook and elastic underneath it. I try it on, turn around in the mirror and take it off again. I'll have to cut the tag off my bra. I can practically read the blue label through the dress. I pick out a decent pair of panties and a slip tight enough not to rumple under the spandex.

I curl my hair and spray it stiff. My blonde curls bounce on my shoulders, my bangs dance high on my forehead—and my dress creeps up my thighs. I apply my makeup. Each time I lift an arm, the dress on that side takes a hike up my leg. I stand on my tiptoes and try to see it in the bathroom mirror. I pull the hem back down to meet the top of my knees. I take a deep breath. Even that movement pulls the dress up. I go up the stairs to show her. Maybe she will make me take it off.

"Well, it looks like it fits you," she says.

It fits? "Yeah, thanks a lot, Mom." *She thinks it fits?* "It's really nice."

I haven't seen myself in a full-length mirror yet, so I go over to the front hall closet to make sure my slip and underwear aren't too obvious underneath.

Yikes! There is no underneath. Just the walk up the stairs has shimmied my slip up past my hips, bunching it around my waist. The dress is not much lower than my crotch. The spandex stretches in sexy horizontal lines over my thighs. I reach under the skirt to pull the slip back down. I run my hands down my waist to smooth the dress back to my knees. *This is going to be a long night.*

I practice breathing lightly in front of the mirror. Short breaths don't lift it quite as much. I tuck in my tummy. *Okay, that helps a little.* I stand straight so the dress won't lift up over my bum. I look at it from the left, the right, over my shoulder. I try walking. Maybe if I take baby steps. I try a mincing walk. *Oh, crap, this is just terrible.* The phone rings in the front hall, and I answer it.

"Hello?"

"Hi, it's me." *Shawna.*

"Are you coming?"

"Yeah, my dad says he'll drive us." I am squirming in the full-length front hall mirror. The doorbell rings, and Mom calls out from the kitchen. "Come in."

"Great, I'll be ready when you get here. What are you wearing?"

"My new sweater and black skirt. What are you wearing?"

"A white dress Mom got me." I pull and smooth and twist to see my behind.

"A new dress? Lucky!"

"Yeah."

"See ya."

"Okay. See ya in a minute."

I hang up the phone and turn to go downstairs, but then I notice Cory, an adult friend of the family, standing in the doorway. I look at his face, but he's not looking at mine. Mom comes around the corner and sees him seeing me from behind. She steps between us. I shiver and go downstairs quickly to recheck the dress and spray my hair one more time. I hear Mom laughing and animated. I hear Cory, timid and friendly, the way he always is. I come back up the stairs just as Mom closes the door behind him. She waits a moment to be sure he is well down the walk and then turns on her heel, turns on me.

"Well, look at the little slut. Prancing around in her pretty, sleazy little dress."

Mom. Regular Mom now, dark and vicious. Happy, spendy, friendly, laughing Mom has skipped off.

I brace myself for an onslaught. Yelling I can take. As long as the abuse is just words. Hurtful enough. *Just please, please, don't hit me.*

"What were you doing standing there in front of him like that?"

"In front of who? Oh, Cory? Like what?"

"You know what you were doing. I saw him looking at you. I saw him."

"What?"

"You sleazy little bag, you think every man wants you. You think they all want you. You aren't the only good-looking thing in this house. I was cute, too, y'know. And I was cuter than you. Look at those thick hips, that, that . . . that big nose. You are so cocky. You think you are so smart. Just wait till you get married. You'll be fat like me. I was cute, too, y'know."

I'm paralyzed by fear, crying without making a sound. I see myself in the hall mirror. My mascara runs with the tears. The black watercolour stains my cheeks and pools in the creases of my nose. *Why is she doing this to me?*

I want to ask her outright, Why are you doing this? I didn't want that old man to look at me. I feel dirty knowing he even looked at me in this dress. I didn't want that. And if you knew about my hips, why did you buy this awful dress? But I can't. I hold my tongue and remain submissive. I can't win this moment, and she won't lose it at any cost. She didn't buy the dress for me. She bought it for herself, the girl she wishes she was. "Well, stop blubbering and get cleaned up. You look so ugly when you cry. I mean it, stop screwing up your face and get washed. Your friends are going to be here to pick you up."

But she doesn't say, Change out of that slutty, sleazy dress.

I want out of the dress. But I can't change my clothes without her order. If I don't wear it, I won't be going.

So I wear it and spend the evening in the bathroom, tugging it down and trying to hide my hips. She was right. I feel every bit as slutty as she says I am, and men are looking at me.

14

I spent as much time away from home as I could in twelfth grade. I went to early morning classes, after-school clubs, a tutoring job with elementary kids, young women's church activities, and a part-time job at McDonald's, all to keep me busy and away from Mom.

Funny. So many kids get involved in so many activities, and the teachers all think it's a matter of public service and overachieving. I wonder now how many were like me, just trying to find reasons to stay away from home. It didn't matter, though. She would catch me as I passed by, on my way to an activity or when I was trying to get out the door for school without a scene.

"Did you get your report card today?" She is in the kitchen and I am trying to get down to my bedroom unseen.

"Oh, yeah, I did." *Here it comes.*

"Let's see it."

I slump my bag on the table and dig into it, pulling out the sheet with my mid-term marks on it. The grades are good, some even fantastic—except for one, the one she goes to.

"Looks like you are pretty stupid in math," she says. "Pull up your socks and start working at it, Autumn, or you'll be flunking out."

"I got ninety-seven in English and ninety-two in biology."

"Yeah, what happened to the other eight percent, eh?" she sneers. She goes into her glare. Boring into my eyes with hers, daring me to speak another word, just daring me. I start to walk away. But I stop at the top of the stairs. With the dining room table between us, I feel safe. I can get to my room before she can get to me.

I take her dare. Loudly.

"What the hell's the matter with you?" Louder. "Can't you say anything nice?" It's a page out of her own book. Pure rant. "Can't you see I'm doing everything I can to please you?" Faster. "I can't win. I'll never be good enough for you." Shrieking. I get ready to run if I have to. I don't. Dad appears in the hallway. I didn't know he was home. He is shocked. He's heard me on a rant before, but never against Mom. I see he's speechless. So I let her have the rest of it. "You are a total bag. I hate you. I hate you." Loud. Fast. Shrill.

She does not care. She mocks me. She makes the words with her mouth but does not speak them: I'll never be good enough for you. She laughs out loud. Dad just stands there. I'm surprised. He doesn't take her side.

But I don't care about him either. I'd like to hit her. I want to throw something. But I can't. So I run away. I run down the stairs and slam the door. I toss my body onto my bed. I scream into my pillow and heave and hit and blow snot all over my sheets. Until I sense the door opening. Now I'm going to get it. I whirl on my bed.

Dad stands in my doorway. *Take my side, not hers.* I stop screaming and start crying. Screams for her; tears for him.

"Autumn." He's going to take her side. I hear it in his voice.

"I can't live with her any more, I am scared to go near her, I can't do anything right and she hates me. She really hates me."

"Just give her a break," he says, keeping his voice low. So she can't hear him? He's afraid of her, too? "She's having a rough time right now." He is. He's afraid.

"Right now? She's having a rough time all of the time. Rough times don't look like this. This is crazy."

Dad reaches over to my wall and pulls my cartoon calendar from its nail. "Look, read this cartoon." I take the calendar and look at the monthly joke about PMS.

"Wha . . ."

"It is called PMS," he says.

I sit up and spit the words, "This is not PMS. PMS does not last all month." *Or all year. Year after year after year.* Some of my friends have tiffs with their moms, too, but not like this. Other moms are not like her. He cannot excuse this abuse and call it PMS. He can't. He just can't.

He turns to leave. "Someday you'll understand."

Never. I'll never understand her.

15

"**M**om! Mom, are you home?" I know she is. At least one of her is. I see her shoes and purse. I need permission, so I need Skippy Mom today. "Mom?" The house is dark, the blinds all drawn. The kitchen counter is strewn with Sprite, Orange Crush, and Mountain Dew cans and Popsicle wrappers. So. The kids made their own lunches today. They are out to play. I saw Dad leave with the little ones.

"Mom? I need to ask you. Can I go with Shawna?" I am sixteen but I have to ask.

No reply.

So I look for her. On hot days like today, she keeps cool with drawn shades and blowing fans. I hope she's not asleep.

I check the hall. The boys' room. The bunk beds, top and bottom. Sometimes she naps in their room.

"Mom?"

Her bedroom door is ajar. I push it open. The room is dim. She's pulled the blinds with the tassels and fringe that swing when the fan blows over them on each pass. My eyes adjust. There!

In the big grey La-Z-Boy chair chair. Asleep. I shuffle into the dim and tap her. But it's not her after all, just lumps of clean laundry. I catch my reflection in the tall mirror set atop the wide, low dresser. It's me, tall and thin now. And bleached blonde and tan. I'm not ugly any more. My peach knit tank top makes my tan look darker than it really is. I look good and . . . "Oh!" Another face peeks over my shoulder.

No. It's only Jesus, his life-sized portrait over the bed. Mom is not here.

"Mom, where are you?"

I have a sense about this now.

She's playing a new game. Maybe trying to see if I'll go without asking.

Is she watching me right now?

I creep to the master bathroom. I slide the door into its pocket in the wall. It's dark. She's not here.

I turn away. I holler, "Mom! C'mon, I just want to go to Shawna's."

If this is a game, it's not a fun one.

She was here only half an hour ago. She was agitated, mean. Dad took the kids away because of her. She's here; I know it.

"Mom?"

I leap down the stairs three at a time and breeze through the bedrooms, bathroom, the family room, the kitchenette, the laundry room. All the regular places to hide in our house.

Okay, so she's not hiding out in the regular places. I've played hide-and-seek in this house. I know all the best places. I step down into the space under the garage floor. The cold storage room. A single bulb casts long shadows into the gloom. The walls are lined with endless shelves of canned goods and emergency supplies. Wrapping paper. Boxes of clothes. No Mom.

I hate her games. Back up the stairs, two at a time, I slam through the screen door to the backyard. *I'm out of time.*

Shawna and her family will go without me. But I have to ask. The last time I left without asking, I paid with a bloody nose. Mom met me at the front door. Not a word. Just a smack on the face. I'm not ugly any more. I can't let her mess up my face.

I have time to make one more sweep. It's scary. I know she knows I'm looking. Looking behind furniture, under beds. She's waiting to spring out at me, thinking she is so funny. I just know she is here. But I'll be a good sport. When she's done laughing, I'll ask. She'll let me go if I'm a good sport, if I act amused at her little game.

"Mom, where are you? C'mon. Please?" Nothing.

I stand in the hall, defeated. I'll have to give up and call Shawna. Tell her to go on without me.

"Dang it, Mom, where are you?"

I remember a time when she boasted her closet was so big she could fit in it easily. I can make one more quick pass at her room.

I slide the door open and jump back at a flash of movement. I let out a little yip. Mom? No. A silky gown drops off the hanger.

Ridiculous. This is just ridiculous.

I brace my hand on the bathroom door as I stoop to pick up the nightgown. I brace my hand on . . .

The door?

The pocket door is shut.

But I left it open. I stand up. This is like a movie, and not a funny one. Now I am afraid. She's behind that door.

I've been all over the house looking for her. Now I don't want to find her.

I should go. Pretend I was never looking for her. I should go, but I can't fake it now. I've been calling her name all over the house. She'll know I was looking. I'm too scared to try the door. So I knock.

"Mom, are you in there?" Silence.

"Mom, I just want to go to Shawna's house." Silence.

I push one of her buttons. "Dammit, Mom, if you're in there, just say I can go."

She's not. She would have yelled back at me: Don't you dare talk like that. Or, Get over here so I can soap out your mouth. I turn to leave.

Mmph.

A sound.

I stop.

I know I heard a sound.

There is silence now, but I heard something. I know I did. I'm scared and this is stupid. I take a breath and slam open the door.

Nothing.

It is dark. Good. Okay, I was wrong. Not here. That was my own sound, my own whimper. I give myself a weak smile. Not here. I'm so dumb. I turn to go. A chill catches me by the neck. A voice speaks from the back of my head.

She's in the shower.

My Girl has decided to join me in full voice now.

No.

Yes, in the shower. You know she is. No use denying it.

My Girl has a knack for showing up at the times when I need her most, even when I don't want her advice.

Don't be such a chicken. Just open the shower and get it over with.

"Mom?"

In the soft glow from under the bedroom window shade I can make out the handle for the shower door. I snap it open.

She's in my face. The killer in *Psycho*, only *in* the shower instead of outside it.

I wince away.

Right there. Face to face. Ackk!

"Mom. What . . . ? You scared me—"

She pulls back from me, too, but I am the more horrified. There she stands, my mother, fully dressed, cowering in her dark shower stall. Her hands are close to her face and her eyes are wide open like a terrified kitten's, a ghoul's.

That look!

"Mom?"

"Don't call me Mom. Don't call me Mom. Don't call me Mom. Don't call me Mom." The face says she is terrified. And yet . . . and yet she is . . . smirking?

"Mom, come out of there. Please?" *This is so sick.*

"Don't call me Mom. Don't call me Mom."

"Aw, come on, come out of there, *please*." She's right about one thing. This is not any of my moms. Not Dark and Dangerous Mom. Not happy, Skippy, Spendy Mom. Not even Blank Mom. This is nothing but . . . Sicko Mom.

Dad is gone and I am alone with her and she is sick and I am terrified. "Mom, what—?"

"Just get out!" That's more like it, more like herself, just a glimpse of Dark and Dangerous Mom. "Get out of here, just get the hell out of here."

I do.

I leave her in the dark, shaking and so . . . sinister. Worse than she's ever been.

Get out, she said. *Permission enough.*

I close all the doors, the shower, the bathroom, the bedroom, the front hall, the grand entryway. I walk out into the street. My feet tell me to run away, but I keep them to a brisk walk. I feel the sun on my face, warm, comforting, relaxing, trying to ease the knots in my jaws.

Before, when weird stuff happened in our house, we dared not talk about it. Mom called it "airing our dirty laundry for the neighbours." Dad called it "infidelity." It would be pure disrespect to say that Mom wasn't acting well. So I never did. But this? This was more than not acting well.

This is why they taught me so well. The denial, fidelity, the warped sense of honour. This is the darkest of the dark secrets they keep from me. This secret isn't mine to tell. It isn't even mine to acknowledge.

So I walk away. I walk down our street to the end, where a path begins and curves sharply to the left. No secrets here in the great bright white windy out-of-doors. Nothing like the dank, dim hole where I left my mother.

Up the little hill and over the rise, take a right-hand turn at the Y. Right to Shawna's. Shawna and I go shopping and buy shoes with our McDonald's wages. Then I stay over for a summer barbecue in the backyard. I watch Shawna's mom bustling about the meal, her dad at the barbecue. We sit on the patio and drink lemonade and laugh until the sun goes down. This is how a family is supposed to act. This is normal.

Unlike Mom. Huddled, hiding, trembling. Nuts. *My mother is nuts.* I try the words inside my head. *My mother is a lunatic. My mother is mad.*

Would Shawna believe me if I said it aloud? No.

She's mad at you? Again? For what?

No, Shawna, she's insane. Crazy. Nuts. Bananas. Mental.

Shawna: *Well, my mom gets pretty extreme, too. Everybody freaks out sometimes.*

No, Shawna wouldn't get it. No one would. Today I found her in the shower like some wide-eyed monster . . .

Forget about disrespect or infidelity. I can never tell anybody about what went on inside my house. I am too ashamed.

And not just about Mom.

I am ashamed and afraid for me, too. That when I feel sad, the light shrinks in my room. That when I am really sad, even the sun goes dark. That the world is an enemy some days, often many days on end. That I am evil. That my reflection in the mirror is the devil. Not today, but some days.

That the monster I found hiding in the shower today is me.

16

Every teen is a monster in one way or another, and maybe that's why nobody called me on my own bad behaviour. They might have called it raging hormones, teen angst, confusion, frivolity, stupidity. They might have thought I was drunk or high. No one ever called me crazy. But I was. And dangerous.

Far from being the scrawny recluse of just a few years past, I would flirt with anyone, including teachers—my third block teacher, in particular. I would tease him with a brush on the neck, my fingers across his hand on the desk, questions about private tutoring—game playing, pure and simple—and My Girl would scream: *Stop it, don't be a fool, you don't want this, you don't mean it. You are going to get hurt.*

I didn't believe My Girl until the teacher stopped me in the hall.

"Miss Stephan."

"Huh?"

I turn from my friends, a pack of girls with bag lunches and binders, laughing and teasing each other in a circle, flipping hair and shifting weight from one hip to the other, animated, young, energetic, coy, good girls wanting to be oh so bad. He is in the doorway. I was very bad yesterday myself.

Oh, no. My Girl sees it in his eyes before I do.

"Mr. Purdue, did you call me?"

"Miss Stephan, do you have a minute for me?"

My friends stop giggling to listen in. I don't want to go to him. I know I was flirtatious, but . . . am I in trouble or what? *I told you to stop. I warned you. Now you are going to get it.*

I clutch my binder to my chest with both arms and move toward him. I hear the girls whisper and titter behind me. Mr. Purdue grins and ushers me into the classroom.

"I've been thinking about you."

"Oh?" *Uh-oh*.

"Just wondering if you have some time after school. For some lessons?"

"Well, I have Student Council meeting." *Just say no*.

"After that, Autumn. You need me. Just a little tutoring." He smiles and puts his hand on the wall, shifting his weight, leaning into my space.

"I can't." *You can't play like that, you idiot. I told you.*

"I don't need help with your class, Mr. Purdue. My grades are fine."

He leans out of my space. I am not the girl I was yesterday. Yesterday I would have raised my eyebrow and laughed: I'll be there. Or wet my lips: What's the subject? Or dropped my binder and stooped low to give him a peek.

I'm not that girl today. He is confused, but he gives it a second go.

"Autumn, I'm offering you a little one-on-one, if you want it." He looks in my eyes, at my mouth, and back to my eyes.

I am stone cold.

He tries to break the chill. "Only if you want it."

You don't. Say you don't want it and get out of here.

"I've got an eighty-eight average in your class. I don't think I need any tutoring."

The red was in his neck before I finished. I walked around him, my heart pounding into my binder. I passed my girlfriends in the hall. "Hey, Autumn—?"

Next day I went to the school counsellor.

"I want to drop my third block class."

"Why?"

"No reason. I just want a spare in that time block."

"I can't let you do that. You're on Student Council, and we need you to be a good example for the rest of the class."

"I can't go back."

"Why?"

"I can't tell you." I cry hard and the counsellor waits, but I don't offer more.

"If you won't tell me what the problem is, then I can't help you."

"And I can't tell you."

I skipped every third block for the rest of the semester, and the office never bothered to call me on it. I studied the textbook and wrote the final exam. I was hoping for a miracle—like high school credits from heaven—but no. I failed the course with a mark of twenty-six. I didn't care. Mr. Purdue didn't come back to school the next semester.

I was brutal with boys, too.

My Girl worked overtime trying to keep me in line. She knew things she wouldn't tell me. When I got too close to any boy, she would step in to give me half a memory and a bad feeling. I told Shawna about the effect one boy had on me.

"Shawna, I didn't mean to hurt him. But when he kissed me good night, I just wanted to puke."

"Did he have bad breath?"

"No, no, it's not like that. When guys get too close or if they kiss me, I get this vomit feeling."

"Gross, like a flu or what?"

"No. I don't know, I can't name it. It's like being in a cold, wet bathing suit in front of a room full of dry, sarcastic boys."

"Sick," said Shawna. "That's a feeling to avoid."

So I tried. I became Cinderella. When the clock struck, I bolted. I ran home, never to go back.

The first major player in my game was Brian, a twenty-two-year-old with shoulder-length hair, a thick tongue, and a big truck. *How do you like this one, Mom?* Turned out he wasn't worth the shock value. Under the big truck and the long hair was a wimpy kid with no ambition. He was stupid to boot. And whiny. I told him to stop calling. He didn't let go easily. He fell all over himself with flowers and poetry and teddy bears. I didn't know what to do. I hadn't yet learned the art of breaking up. But I picked up on that skill pretty quickly.

Orly seemed okay until he kissed me. His lips were fat, wet, inside-out lips. Troy was good-looking and never whiny, but we went to a party and he made a joke about me to his friends, and I felt ashamed and small. Tyler lasted long enough to make me want to commit to him, but one night he kissed me too hard. I never saw him again. He even called my dad to ask if he knew what went wrong. Dad was sympathetic. He tried to make me talk to Tyler. I didn't.

I'd graduated high school by now, so I packed up and moved to Edmonton. Mostly to avoid Tyler.

I came home two months later when a boy named Derek dragged me off my path of destruction. Derek was my first angel. I'm sure God put him in my life to save me from myself. He was rational, intelligent, and kind. He had known me only for a week or so when he told me he was taking me back home to my parents. I didn't argue. I needed someone to take charge of me. In the two months I had lived away from home, I had gone through two roommates and two jobs. I was seventeen and I couldn't make sense of anything in my world. Derek made sense, so for that week, he became my world.

He drove me back to Fort McMurray to drop me off. I was wild, bold, loud, and obnoxious. My Girl was embarrassed. *Shut up*, she told me.

But I didn't, and before Derek left me in Fort McMurray, I sat the whole lot of them down at the kitchen table. Mom, Dad, and Derek. I announced that Derek and I were getting married. *Shut up.* I said I knew Derek was the one because of the size of his nose. *Shut up. I told you.* I told them I was not attracted to him at all, and that is why God wanted me to be with him. *Oh, please, Autumn, stop it. Don't be so rude. You sound crazy. Just shut up.*

Derek didn't think we were meant for each other, and neither did Mom and Dad. Derek politely excused himself and drove the six hours to his home. My first angel never came back. Boy after boy I teased and taunted and ran away from. I came so close to self destruction, but I reserved the best part of me. Not because I was good, but because I had no say. I was a virgin for two good reasons. First, Mom. She taught me, bold and clear, that there was only one place for sex. Only within the covenant of marriage. I know plenty of kids are taught that way, and that logic is only enough to carry a very few through the temptation, but

Mom was different, so full of conviction. And when the knowledge of my mother's conviction wasn't enough to keep me out of trouble, there was always a backup: a fragmentary vision of me in a flannel nightgown. Standing on my head. Then the choking, disgusting, terrifying feeling of bathing in my own vomit, bits of curvy pasta and corn and chunks of hamburger bobbing on the water. Every boy I got close to made me queasy. Even the good boys could make me puke.

17

I had been gone for only two months, but my bedroom had already been taken over by Daniel. He had been sharing rooms all his life, and now he was twelve and desperate for his own space. I couldn't take it back from him, so I moved into the laundry closet in the hall. The closet was half the length of my body, but I could easily curl into the fetal position to pull my legs in. I slept on the floor under a shelf and when I decided not to come out, no one noticed. I lay on the floor, getting up only for bathroom breaks, living in a ball on the floor of the closet for a week and a half. I cried and moaned and slept the days away, content to be absorbed in the dark of the mood, giving in to the thick blanket of sleep and sadness that I could not escape and didn't want to avoid.

Then one morning the light turned back on in my head and I came out of the closet. I moved out of Mom's house for a week until I got sick of Shawna's basement and came home. Mom said if I would stay home and help out, I could have a bedroom again. I came home. I cut off my shoulder-length blonde hair, leaving it rough-cut, short, and dyed black.

I went wild. During the day I worked at the city dump as a security guard and weigh-scale operator, and at night I played the dating game. I had no loyalty and no sense. And I chose dangerously. It wasn't fun to choose beggars any more. Now they were mean—the kind of men who hit girls, or grabbed them hard and shoved them against walls, or leaned over in the car and pushed on their throats to make them stop nagging.

I spent New Year's Eve with one of these. And on New Year's Day I nursed my bruise and vowed never to see Ken again. Except to give him back his leather jacket. Then I would never see him again. I went to give him back the jacket. He threw it back in my face. He said he'd see me in a week. That I'd better come to my senses. That I'd better not call him before the week was up, because he'd be on the prowl.

That night Shawna inherited a great leather jacket.

Now I spent my days sitting in the trailer at the weigh scale at the dump watching the trucks filled with stench drive on and off. I wrote prose and poetry and begged God for help.

So God sent me help in the form of a small man with thinning hair and a hot car. Jon, my second angel, didn't want to date me. He was too smart for that. He did drive me around in his car and lecture me. He said he'd even pay me to grow up. "A hundred bucks if you can go three months without a boyfriend."

So I did. All I needed was for someone to tell me to do it. I wrote off men for three months. At the end of it, he took me to lunch. I forgave him the hundred bucks. It wasn't the money I needed.

"Thanks, Jon."

"So what's next for you?"

"I don't know. I've been working for my dad and I think I'm going to go to school. My friend Greg is coming back from the Philippines in a year. He's the kind of guy I'd like to marry. He never let me run over him the way other guys do. And he never hurt me."

"Yeah, a year is good—but you're way too young to think about marriage."

I swore off dating again. Three months gave me enough time to see the patterns in my life. My moods were like the ocean tides. Either high or low or moving toward high or low. Never stable. Always pulsing and throbbing. The sparkler state of mania. Or the dark flannel depression.

"Your father is having an affair."

"What?"

Mom and I are parked in the church parking lot, slouching in the bucket seats of the van, eating chocolate bars. I sit up straight and turn to face her. "You're not serious."

"I am. I've known it for a long time."

"He's never alone with anyone, Mom. Not anyone. Not even Shawna when she needs a ride home. How could he be?"

"Oh no. It's not sexual. He'd never do that. It's an affair of the heart, and that's worse."

"Is this what you have been fighting about?" I have heard her lately, it seems every night, slamming and stomping and ranting in the bedroom. Their after-hours affair is not a dance any more. It is a rumble through the floorboards, the sound of breaking glass and breaking hearts and broken promises. And I don't want to be here in the van to hear about it from her.

Mom cries and chews on the chocolate and I do my best to console her. When we are done and I am thoroughly confused, she drives home. She gets out of the van, and Dad meets her halfway down the driveway. She brushes past him, and before I can get out, he is in the driver's seat.

"Let's go," he says, and pulls out of the driveway. *Oh no.*

"Dad, I . . ."

"What did she say to you?"

"Dad, no."

"Autumn, you have to help me here. What did she say?"

"She says you're cheating on her."

"What? No. Not this again." Dad pulls over and covers his face with his arm.

"Again?"

"Aww, she does this, this accusation thing. Every once in a while she just gets almost paranoid. I can't convince her that I'm faithful, and she can't make any sense or talk to me about it, and then one day she just forgets about it and we move on. Dammit, I can't believe we're back to this again. Does she think I'm really cheating?"

"She—"

"I go way out of my way, Autumn. I do everything I can to avoid even looking suspicious. Why can't she trust me? You have to talk to her. You have to talk some sense into her." He's not crying, but he looks as if he's going to puke, and I can't bear to see him like this. Dear Dad, so clumsy in relationships, so desperate to make Mom believe that he loves her.

"I'll try."

I did try. I failed, and their problems felt like my problems, and nothing got better. If anything, the situation grew worse. Mom was vengeful and angry. She became bold and critical of Dad at the dinner table and bad-mouthed him to the kids. Dad gave up trying to convince her of his innocence. He became sick with a rare flu strain that flattened him. Now he was not in his office or at the church. He was at home on the couch, twenty-four hours a day. Day after day after day. And still she was not satisfied.

"He'll get his," she said.

We were standing in the kitchen, and she was on again. A rant out of the blue. "He'll know how this feels, to be betrayed."

"Mom."

"He's in love, it's an affair of the heart. We can all do that, you know. We can all find a soulmate."

I had to get away, and not just to bed or to my job. Shawna and I drove around the province visiting friends and shopping and acting like girls. As we travelled, we called on old friends and parents of friends to put us up for the night. My mother drove me out of the house and into a man's arms. Her paranoia brought Dana to me, of all things. Dana. My blessing, her curse. Her curse and entirely her own doing.

It was March and we were restless. Shawna and I decided to take a road trip to visit friends twelve hours south. We left in the morning and planned to stay at Greg's parents' place, halfway to Calgary. When the snow came and the storm blew in, we were stuck. Our little car barely limped into the city, and then we were grounded, with no way to go until the roads cleared. So we hung out with Greg's parents and his older sister, Jennifer.

"You might as well have fun while you're here." Greg's mother was so sweet.

Jennifer invited a couple of guys over to the house to play games and eat and listen to music. I didn't recognize the names and I didn't really care who was coming. I didn't put on my makeup, I didn't curl my hair. I wore green corduroy overalls and a white T-shirt and I was relaxed. This was not a party. This was not about impressing anyone or pretending anything. This was just about having fun on a stormy night with friends. I wasn't looking for more.

Jennifer, her friend Stacey, Shawna, and I are sitting at the kitchen table when the doorbell rings. *The boys.* Jennifer hops up from the table and goes around the corner, down the stairs, to open the door.

"Hi, guys, come on in."

The first boy speaks: "Thanks, it's cold out there."

Then the second boy: "Yeah, it's cold. What are you doing dragging us out in this kind of weather?" Then he laughs.

It's him. My Girl speaks up.

It's him.

What?

You are going to marry that boy.

I have heard her many times when I have met boys, but I have never listened and I'm not going to start now. Especially now that My Girl is crazy. I haven't even seen this guy's face and already she has decided I am going to marry him. *Right.*

Jennifer comes up the stairs followed by the two boys.

"Okay, Autumn and Shawna, this is Hugh and Dana."

"Hi."

"Hi."

"Hi."

"Hi." *It's him. Autumn, pay attention. This is him.*

Shut up.

She doesn't. I scoot over to the middle chair, leaving one on my left empty. Dana sits down and Hugh takes a seat next to Shawna. I turn to look at Dana while we talk about my car and the storm and what did I think I was doing, driving from Fort McMurray to Calgary in the middle of a spring snowstorm? I study him. Dana is blond, clean-cut, with fair skin, dimpled but ruddy, masculine. When he sits next to me, he takes up space. Broad shoulders, big hands. Thick neck.

I like him. Not because My Girl says so. Because he is funny. Calm, reserved, intelligent. He laughs about his missionary experience in Japan, his high school graduation in Pakistan. He travelled the world before he turned nineteen, but he has grown up in southern Alberta close to my acreage, Mom's garden. He knows my roots. And My Girl starts picking at me.

Why didn't you spend a few minutes fixing yourself up before he got here?

Stop it, I tell her. I can't throw myself at him.

You should have worn your makeup and done your hair.

I'm glad I didn't.

You should have worn normal clothes.

These are comfortable.

How will you see him again?

I probably won't.

Tell him you want to, do something. Don't let him leave without a plan to see him.

Shut up.

I wouldn't do it. I was not going to get sucked back into the game. I was done with that. We played stupid games, the kind Mom played at her parties. The first one was a game at the table. One team hid a coin in their fists, and the other team had to guess where the coin was. It meant passing the coin under the table and tricking the other side. Then the fists were brought up and the other team had to guess who had it. Dumb game, but I wasn't thinking much about it. Or about anything after the first time he touched me—on the palm of my hand as he slipped a coin to me. I was baptized with electricity. I felt his touch everywhere. This I had never experienced before. This I knew was different. This I could not wreck.

I told you.

He must have felt it, too. He touched my hand under the table more often than he passed me the coin.

We had fun at Greg's house. We goofed around and told stories, and before he went home, we lay on the carpet and he used his finger to draw a map to the church, pushing the roads and stoplights into the mat of soft grey.

We planned to see each other at church the next day, but didn't. Just as well because I was going to have to snub him. I decided after he left that I was not going to play my games on him. I didn't want to hurt him. He was different. He deserved better.

18

Shawna and I went to Fort McMurray, and I was sure I had seen the last of Dana. But I had to go back to Edmonton to take college entrance exams. I ended up going down two days early with Mom and Dad because Dad was still sick and needed to get some tests done in the university hospital.

The hotel is so boring. Two days to kill off before my exam. Two days alone with Mom and Dad. I can't stand the quiet. I can't sit still. So I get up my nerve and call Dana.

"There's a hockey game on."

"I know, I'm watching it."

"The hotel has a big screen TV in the lounge. We could watch it here?"

"Okay, I'll be over at intermission." That makes me smile. He doesn't dump the hockey for me. Very Canadian. Very grounded.

Later we watch second- and third-period hockey and talk and laugh. He doesn't try to kiss me. I'm glad. We go to the games room to play ping-pong. He wins. We play pool, and he wins again. He doesn't let me beat him. And he tells me I owe him a dinner besides. So we agree to have dinner tomorrow night. He'll pick me up at six. There is no kissing, but once he puts his hand on my back and I feel it again. Pure electricity. My Girl is happy.

He's so stable, so strong and intelligent. And reserved. He talks and laughs and doesn't try anything else. I should tell him that he's winning my heart. More important, my stomach: *You don't make me feel like puking.*

"Where were you?" Mom is agitated.

"Just down in the games room with Dana Stringam."

"Where is he?"

"He had to go home, he works really early."

"Where?"

"At the car wash."

"The car wash?"

"He's just off a mission for the church. He's going to college in September." I've gone to bed before she can say anything else.

I go to bed, but I don't sleep. I try to make myself stop thinking about him, but every time I am drifting into sleep, My Girl pipes up with a *Good job!* or a *Can you believe it?* I tell her to shut up.

The next morning I'm not happy-skippy-spendy like Mom sometimes gets, but I go shopping anyway, to get out of the hotel and to find something to wear for dinner. I come back with a bag from Sears and a big smile on my face.

"Okay, so let's see what you got." Mom loves shopping. She is on the bed with my limp, sweaty Dad, watching television.

I run to the back of the suite where my bedroom is and get dressed. I choose a casual outfit with floral leggings and a black shirt. It's cute. The other side of the continent from that white spandex of not long enough ago.

"What do you think?"

"Oh, cute pattern, Autumn. I like those leggings."

"Thanks." A compliment? "He's coming in about half an hour, so I have to get ready." She's giving me a compliment? *Something's up.*

I curl my hair and do my makeup. I am putting on my shoes when I hear the knock on the hotel door. *He's here.* I tie my shoes while Mom answers the door. Then she is in my room. She shuffles her feet and kicks at the carpet; she pretends her silky zip-up nightgown has pockets and stuffs her hands deep into them. I stand up to watch her. *Let's have it.* She looks at me looking at her and tucks her chin into her chest.

"Uh, hi, is Autumn there?" Making fun of him.

"Mom."

"Oh, good grief, Autumn, you can do better than that."

"He's really great."

"You can do better. And it's too bad your thighs look so thick in that outfit." She's picking. It's been a long day alone with Dad and no kids to pick at but me.

He's at the door, Autumn, and you're an adult. Just walk away and go to him. Don't let her take him from you. You don't need her permission to be happy. Go now. For once, I listen to My Girl.

"I'll be back later." I brush by her and leave her standing in her gown. "Bye." She has never seen me like that, calm, self-assured. I think it makes her feel small. I think it makes her feel silly. She wants to know if I will choose a guy I have known for a day over my mother of eighteen years.

My Girl tells me: *Whatever it takes, you are not losing this one. Whatever it takes, and if that means Mom is mad, then so be it.*

We spent the evening laughing about his adventures in Pakistan, Rome, and Idaho.

"So, what are your plans?" he asks.

"College in the fall."

"What do you want to take?"

"Dietary Sciences or English."

"You like that stuff?"

"Love it."

"I like a girl with plans."

"Really?" I smile. He likes me. At least he likes my plans. Still, I can't read him. *It's him. You won't be in college because you'll be married. I'm telling you, it's him.*

I dig into another bite of chocolate cake. Dana clears his throat. I look up and he is pursing his lips over his teeth.

"Sorry, but do I have anything in my teeth?" He smiles. He has packed chocolate cake into his gums and over every tooth. The inside of his lips are black and I have to cover my mouth before I spew dessert all over the table. I laugh, and he laughs, and he swallows his cake. "Do I have anything in mine?"

"Yeah, just a piece of pepper on the right . . . you got it."

"Thanks."

He did all that so I wouldn't be embarrassed when I found out I had peppered chicken in my smile?

Dana didn't kiss me after dinner and he didn't kiss me the next day after my exam. He didn't kiss me over our fancy dinner at a French restaurant, although I was wearing a sleek black dress that showed my legs and collarbone. He didn't kiss me at the dance we went to. He danced with me, and then he danced with other girls, and I danced with some boys I knew, and we were both feeling odd about being there. When we met up again, he danced a slow song with me. He held me tight, pressing me to him with one hand on my back and my hand in his. I looked into his eyes. My Girl didn't even have to say it.

"Do you want to go?" Dana asked in my ear.

"Okay."

"There's nobody here," he whispered.

"I know."

"There's nobody here but you."

He didn't kiss me in the car, but he held my hand.

"Hey, Wilma, I could get used to holding your hand." Wilma? I looked at him—he was grinning—and then I looked at my narrow hand in his huge fist. I started to giggle and he finished the joke. "Just call me Fred." I got it: *The Flintstones*.

We laughed as he drove to the Legislature grounds. We got out and walked down the path in the trees and out onto the bridge where the night wind blew off the icy North Saskatchewan River, pinking our noses and stinging our cheeks. We stood and laughed and talked about everyday things. I pulled my jacket around me. He took my shoulders and looked me in the eyes.

"Are you cold?"

"Hardly." How could I be when he was looking at me like that?

He kissed me. *Finally*. And again.

"I'm glad you're here with me," he said.

"Me, too." *Wow, you don't make me want to puke*.

I knew that I would never be the same again. It was the ninth of April.

19

Dana was not a game player, and I could not turn him into one. As the mood tide rose, I grew sick. I couldn't hide my inner struggle from him.

We are on our way to a beach, and I am glazed over with a fury.

"What's the problem, Autumn?"

"Don't know."

"Are you okay? 'Cause I'd like to know why you're so stinking mad."

"I don't know."

"Let's pretend you're not mad at me."

"I'm not."

"Then just tell me how you feel."

I turn to face him. He is driving and trying to look at me at the same time.

"It's just that sometimes I get this feeling, like being naked in a crowd. Like using the toilet in the middle of a fancy restaurant, exposed, y'know? Naked?"

"Do I make you feel like that?"

"No." *Everybody makes me feel like that, eventually.* "Sorry, just forget it. I just get this feeling. It's like everything is distorted, and I can't speak right or hear right. Everything is filtered through this terrible glass box around my head. It's not you. I'm sorry."

"You feel like you're in a glass box?"

"Yes." *Sure, if that's what he understands from what I said, just go with it.*

"You should maybe see a neurologist or something."

Or something. You have no idea.

High tides mean fun, though, and so whatever damage I did in the car, I made up for on the beach. We played beach volleyball and splashed and laughed and ate good food, and he was glad I was there with him after all.

The next week I changed. I stopped talking so much on the phone. I decided not to make the trip to see him for the weekend. I cried on Saturday morning when he called to see if I was coming. I said no, and he drove to me. I was dark and shallow and cold and he didn't understand low tide. He felt me slipping away. Later in the week he called to say he'd be gone for a while. Fine by me.

He came back after a week, different, determined, sure of himself and sure of me. He came back and proposed.

"I want to marry you, Autumn." He is on his knee on the stone steps of the Legislature. It is two in the morning, and the fountains are lit behind him. It is all trees and fountains and flowers and Dana. "I prayed about this. I went away and thought about you and me and I prayed so hard, and I know that you are mine. I know we're young, but we can grow up together. I just know this is right. Will you? Will you marry me?"

It was the second of June when I said yes.

Mom hated Dana. I tried to make her love him, but she refused to take to him because he did not buy into her game. He was a kid too bold, too willing to challenge her on her own greater understanding of the universe. She ranted about the evils of cola and the connection between beverages and the fires of hell, and he laughed. She raged that she was the centre of the universe, that when she left the room we would cease to exist until she returned. He told her to go ahead and leave. "Meet you back here in an hour." Dana didn't play the game. He didn't know that he was supposed to listen and nod and take it all seriously, like the rest of them.

Just one more reason to marry him.

Our August wedding was brutal. Mom ripped her toenail off the night before in a freak toe-stubbing accident. So she was on painkillers. The kind that made her high. In the morning she was belligerent. She stood outside the hotel yelling at Dad and cursing him about something to do with the kids and the car. She caught me staring at her and hollered across the parking lot, "Are you sure you want to do this? Marriage sucks." For the rest of the day she was stuck on her one-note song.

"Don't do it, Autumn."

I am sitting in my wedding dress and veil on an ornate bench in the Bride's Room. She is sitting beside me in a peach lace two-piece dress and her sandals. It's something out of the cartoons, the way her toe sticks out all blue and green and red and bandaged.

"Let's go. I'll walk out with you and you won't have to be embarrassed when you tell him it's off. You can do better, Autumn. Play hard to get. You can do better." Mom's arm is around my neck.

"It's fine, Mom. I'm fine. Please don't talk like this right now."

"C'mon, you and me, let's go. You don't want to marry this guy. You don't. We'll go on a trip, and you can sell the dress. Don't be like me. Don't get married right now."

"It's a little late for this conversation, Mom." *And I'll never be like you. Never.*

The little old lady who helped me dress is standing in the doorway asking if I'm ready. *I am.* We go down the hall. Mom limps on ahead, and I am married to Dana. Autumn Stephan becomes Autumn Stringam.

We stand at the door and kiss and hug the family as they file past us. Brothers and aunts and a friend from Peace River. And there is Dad. He is proud, and his eyes are wet. He reaches for me first, holding me to his chest. He turns to kiss me on the face and says in my ear, "This is all I ever wanted for you. You are blessed, Autumn." He pulls back and holds my arms and kisses me on the forehead, then turns to Dana and shakes his hand and pulls him into a hug. "Good man, Dana. You are a good man." Dad trusts Dana with me. Dad trusts that Dana is a good man, and I feel victorious and relieved because now I am Dana's wife and I'm free. I'm free of Mom. *Or is it that Mom and Dad are free of me?*

I'm eighteen and I am a wife. But my tide will ebb and flow just the same. It will rise to new highs and drop to the lowest of lows. Poor Dana. He has no idea what he's married. We set up house in a furnished basement apartment. It is dark enough to suit the low tide that has swept me off my feet and into bed. Dana thinks I am homesick. But I am just plain sick. My mind is slow and dark, and the bedroom is filthy. We received about thirty towels as wedding gifts, and they are all dirty and all on the floor with all of my clothes and half of Dana's. Dirty tissues spill out of the garbage bin onto the floor by the bed. Cotton balls and shoes and cups and spoons and underwear and newspapers are strewn on the floor, random as a damp dropped salad. It is three o'clock in the afternoon.

My Girl wakes me up. *Dana will be home in half an hour. Get up. Get your act together. It's not so tough to take care of yourself and him. It's not so tough.*

I have to get out of bed before he sees that I have not moved yet today. My bladder is full, but I am not hungry. I stumble into the kitchen and lean on the open utility shelves stocked to the top with Mary Kay makeup, the most recent evidence of a high tide. I was going to sell it all and start a business in Edmonton and win a pink Cadillac. I catch my breath as I look at the dishes. All of them. Every dish in the house is on the countertop, and the stench is awful. I push them around and run dishwater. *Maybe that will fool him.*

I pull out the ironing board and I grab some clothes and lay a shirt over the board. I go in the living room and fluff the pillows and move the magazines and take the cups back into the kitchen.

Twenty minutes and he'll be home. Yeah, I get it.

I bathe, leave my hair dry, shave my armpits. I am in my jeans and back in the kitchen by the time he walks in. Dana smells of cardboard. We couldn't afford school right away, so he got a job at the local box company loading printed cardboard boxes off the cutter and onto the pallets. He is dusty from head to toe. Dust is in his nose, on his skin, in his clothes. And he is thirsty.

"What are you drinking?" I ask as he walks into the kitchen.

"Coke."

"You're drinking Coke?" *Stop now, drop it now. Don't say it, Autumn.*

"Yup. What are you doing?" He sucks on the straw. And my eyes fill with tears. *Oh, here we go . . .* My Girl leans back. She's got the best seat in the house to watch the show she knows is coming.

"I can't believe it. Mom said that if you drink Coke, you'll go to hell, and here you are, and you don't want to be with me at all, do you? I can't live with a man who is going to hell. I can't live with you if you're going to hell."

He takes a long pull on the Big Gulp straw and a long look around the kitchen.

"I think I'm there already." He's seen this mess too many times, and this time he walks out of it.

I am still crying when he comes back two hours later and digs into the cleanup.

"I'm sorry." I drop another load of dirty dishes onto the counter. Dana is standing with his hands in the sink and a heap of clean dishes beside him. He doesn't say anything. "We've been married for three months. If you knew this about me before, would you have married me?"

"Nope."

"Do you hate me?" I start crying again, but this time the tears are real and not manipulative, and he knows it. He turns to hold me with his wet hands. He pulls me close.

"Shhh, but I did marry you, and we're going to be okay. You'll be okay and we'll be okay. I don't hate you. It's only love, babe. Love Only."

He still loves me. Imagine. At last. A turning point in my life that doesn't point the way to hell.

20

My marriage was only as good as my moods. I would have a nightmare. Graphic, emotional, terrifying. I'd wake up horrified or hurt or angry. In my dream Dana was a cheater. In my dream Dana mocked me. In my dream Dana killed me.

So, when he woke up, he had to pay.

"Hon, I didn't hurt you. I never did that stuff."

"I feel like you did and I'm really mad."

"But I didn't. You can't blame me for your dumb dreams."

"It doesn't matter if you did or didn't do it. What matters is how I feel, and I feel like you did, so deal with that."

Not only did Dana have to deal with reality, the known factor in his life, he had to deal with my reality where he was a cheater, a mocker, and a killer. He watched me cycle through depression and mania and he didn't know what he was watching. Dumb dreams, homesickness, immaturity, jealousy, PMS. There was always a name for my behaviour, always an excuse for me. When I cried, he held me, and when I laughed, he laughed with me, and if I tried to pick a fight, he just walked away until my mood changed.

He made sense, but his understanding didn't change the pain or the rejection or the filth in my head. My Girl tried to help. *Just don't talk about it. If you can't say something nice . . .*

New rules for Autumn's head, posted right at the front of my brain. *Don't say things that aren't nice. Just because an idea makes sense to you doesn't make it sensible. Just keep your crazy mouth shut.*

Four months passed and then five. Christmas, New Year's Eve. These were the best celebrations of my life. The laughter never turned bitter. There were no surprise endings to the day, no quick flips to anger or malice or jealousy—at least not from him—and when I did it, he soon forgave me.

We were barely six months married when Dad took the whole family to Mexico. He was in better health now and was back to working hard again. The family lived in an apartment on the beach for three months while Dad worked on establishing his water purification business. Mom home-schooled the kids in the apartment before sending them out to play on the sand or in the pool. It was good for her to be away from Canada. When Dana and I came down to visit, she was happy, even giddy. I hoped it was sincere joy: a relaxed mom having fun in Mexico with her kids.

Mom and Dad arranged for a two-night stay in a fancy hotel for Dana and me. When our stay in the hotel was over, we went to Mom and Dad's apartment to stay with them. There wasn't a lot of room, so we slept in the van in the parking lot and helped with the kids and cooking by day.

Mom and I were in the kitchen frying rice puffs when she launched the baby conversation. I wanted to enjoy this time, to talk and laugh and work the way moms and daughters do. I wanted to tell her secrets and feel safe and giggle and make plans for the party on the beach tonight. I wanted to ask her advice and listen and learn. But I knew better than to expect it. Ever since the day I opened the door to the shower stall and came face to face with a monster, I never really expected anything but what she gave me.

"Okay, so are you pregnant yet?"

"No."

"Why not?"

"Dana doesn't think that we should. You know. I just turned nineteen and we've only been married for seven months."

"Oh, is that what Dana says? Let me tell you something. People who mess around with procreation are evil. You keep this up and you will never have babies. Don't think you can just decide if and when and how. It's not your choice."

Uh-oh. "Mom. Dana and I pray every night together, and I trust his judgment on this." *Please don't say—*

"He's evil."

Arrgh!

"He's evil and uninspired and he's taking you down with him."

I walked away before the screaming started. There would be screaming if I stayed another second.

"Don't walk away from me. I'm still your mother."

"And he's my husband." *Mother. Monster. Amazing how close those two words can be.*

I found Dana on the beach with little Celeste and Jeremy and David. "Get me out of here. I have to get out of here right now."

"Okay. Where do you want to go?"

"Just take me away."

Dana rented a scooter, and we drove away into the real Mexico of huts, dirt floors, and marketplaces with dusty fruit stacked high, next to hanging butchered chickens still feathered and hot slabs of beef, bloody and swarming with flies.

We stopped to buy delicious little loaves of tough bread, the kind you rip with your teeth. They were filled with flavor and texture and the odd bit of grit. We filled the scooter box with cans of pop.

We sat by the ocean on the boulders, and Dana told me stories about Pakistan and its meat markets with the flies and the stench and how the people cooked bread on the side of a fiery sandpit. And how he used to go out on the roof and dance in the warm rain, in his underwear.

We tossed our crusts and watched an army of small crabs emerge from the dank between the rocks. They stole away our leftovers, snipping and snapping at each other. We laughed and told stories until the sun, fuchsia and orange and hot, sank into the sea. I didn't tell him about Mom and the baby talk. We had already decided to try to get pregnant this month and I didn't want to wreck the decision by making it something that Mom demanded.

21

"Mom, guess what! I'm pregnant, and you're gonna be a grandma!"

I had just returned from the doctor's office. I felt scared, but thrilled. I had to share. I had to try to be a normal daughter. It was mid-afternoon, and I woke her up with the call.

She didn't have to try to be a normal mom. "Oh, goody," she said. "I think I might be pregnant, too."

Dana could tell from the look on my face. He waited until I was off the phone, then he sat down on the couch and held me while I cried.

"She's what?"

"No, she's not pregnant. She just didn't want me to have the moment. Anything to make things about her. Why do I even bother?"

"Why *do* you bother? Why not ease her out of your life?"

"I thought that this would make her happy. She was mad at me in Mexico because we were waiting too long to get pregnant. Nothing I do will ever make her love me. What can I do to get her to love me?"

"I'm not sure you ever will," he said.

Building a body for my baby was a challenge. Severe nausea and diarrhea gave way to shakes and fatigue. I was sick. I was weak. We lived in a third-storey apartment with stairs and no elevator. I stayed home most of the time, but when we did leave, Dana had to help me down the stairs. My legs shook on every step, and I held the rail and his shoulder to balance and stay upright.

"I can't do it."

"C'mon, sweetie, there's only one more flight."

"I can't, my legs are burning. I'm on fire. I can't."

"Okay, let's sit and rest here for a bit." We sat on the gritty steps, salted with gravel and dried muck from the bottoms of shoes, and he was so patient. He told me I was the sportiest woman he'd ever met. It was such a lie we both had to laugh.

It seemed all I ever did was complain.

Dana never complained.

But he did have one massive headache. It was an unrelenting pain that stayed with him from morning till night. It made him puke in the morning and it made him go to bed early and toss and grunt all night. He ate Tylenol and Advil like mints, popping three or four or five at a time.

His job at the box plant was heavy labour. He had a stiff neck, too, and we blamed it all on his job.

"It's a brain tumour." That was Mom's diagnosis, over the phone, after I told her Dana's symptoms. "My sister had one when she was twelve, and that is definitely what he has."

"Oh, really? I'll tell him."

"You'd better."

I didn't. Of all the ridiculous notions, a brain tumour.

She'd like it if it was. He would die and I would be widowed. Another failure for Autumn. She'd think: Wow, can she pick them, eh? I told her he was no good. I told her not to marry him.

I was pregnant, so I'd have to move home. She would love that even more, because then my baby would be her baby and she would take over and teach my baby everything I swore I would never tell my children.

Later that night he's in excruciating pain. I drag him to a medicentre. The doctor checks his ears, nose, and throat and finds nothing wrong.

"He's hurting all the time. Could it be a brain tumour?" I ask.

"Well, let's see." The doctor has an English accent and is in a big hurry.

"Can you touch your nose with your eyes closed? Good-good. Can you hold your hands high above your head with your eyes closed? Right-right. Very good, no wavering . . . so there it is then. Not a brain tumour, you see. I rather suspect you are experiencing sinus pain as a result of the dusty environment in which you work. Please take Dristan daily to relieve the sinus pressure. All right then, off with you."

He scribbles a note to himself, shuts the folder, looks sideways at me, and walks out.

"Brain tumour, hon?" Red is rising from Dana's neck into his chin and cheeks. "Why would you ask that?"

"Well, Mom said."

"Hey, hon, leave your mom out of this. Brain tumour. Yeah, right."

My Girl agrees. *Ridiculous.*

Dana never raised his voice, never embarrassed me in front of the doctor or anyone else. I'd only know he was upset when he reached the *hon* in a sentence. "See, *hon*, that was a total waste of the evening. I could have been in bed."

Five general practitioners, a chiropractor, and an internal specialist later, we still had no answer for Dana's pain. Dana took his Dristans, Tylenols, and Advils. They might as well have been mints for all the good they did.

In May the pain increased. Now Dana only worked and slept, and he puked as much as I did. His neck was so stiff that he couldn't turn to talk to me without turning his whole body. And he couldn't talk for long because moving his jaw moved his neck and that made him vomit with the pain.

22

When I was five months pregnant, Dana and I drove the five hours to see my mom and dad back in Fort McMurray. Dana brought his headache, and I dragged my bloated body. Before the weekend was over we were in hospital. Dana lay hooked to multiple monitors in an ICU room, and I sat holding my mother's hand and listening to a doctor stumble over telling me the worst possible news.

"A brain tumour?" I whisper.

The doctor calls it something else.

"A brain tumour?" I say it again, staring at the CT scan.

He winces and nods. Not the technical term, mind you, but if that's what you want to call it . . .

I turn to Mom. *You were right?* She nods.

I am reeling. This is some mega-bad dream.

"It's about the size of a mandarin orange," the doctor says. "It's located in the middle of the brain at about temple level." He points at the pictures, outlining the blob with the blunt end of his pen. As if I can't see the mass that blots out the centre of the scan.

I look to Mom. She gives a solemn, smug smile. *I knew it all along, Autumn Dawn, months ago. Okay, so it just took you time to catch up with me and my superior understanding of the universe.*

The doctor interrupts Mom's smile. "We'll get him back to Edmonton. They have a great neurosurgeon there."

We spent a week lying around the hospital in Edmonton, waiting for surgery. We played cards and ordered take-out Chinese and pizza and worked on puzzles and watched television. I was getting bigger while

Dana was getting smaller. He lost a lot of weight during that week, and by the time he was ready for surgery, he looked like a skinny little boy.

Reality hit the night before the operation. The surgeon came in to discuss the risk and potential results of the surgery. Personality change, paralysis, impotence, deafness, blindness, long-term memory loss, brain damage, and death all made the list. Not to mention cancer.

They told me a dozen possible ways that I could lose him. And then a dozen more. It took only one to put me on the edge of panic. I could actually lose my Dana. We signed the papers and acted brave, but I looked at him through different eyes for the rest of the evening. Before we said good night, the rest of the family excused themselves from the room and left Dana and me alone.

We prayed together. A little more desperately than usual and a lot more sincerely. I said the prayer and Dana cried. We felt peace together. But peace didn't stop the tears. I got off my knees and sat by Dana on the bed and cried into his shoulder.

"I need you. You are the only person in my life who has loved me so well. You can't leave me, you just can't. I'll die without you. I will."

"You won't die. You'll live and you'll be happy again and marry a good guy who will treat you the way I do."

"I won't. I won't ever be with another man. I will love you forever, and if you go, I will wait my whole life to be with you again."

I meant it, and he could see that I did. I meant it with every piece of me. Dana was my only love. My gift from God. The kindest person I had ever known. Trustworthy and honest, hardworking and strong and good. And if he went away, I would never live again.

That night, my mother climbed into bed with me. She must have heard me crying. At first I wanted to move away, but then I felt it, the comfort of a mother. I remembered it from when I was small, when she was calm and beautiful and graceful. I felt the comfort of the mom who lay on her bed and shared her dream and made me believe that God lives and that Jesus is the Christ. The mom who made me believe that for one brief moment I was worth loving. She put her arms around me and rocked me to sleep. I let her. It was the last time she showed that she loved me. I thank God for the moment.

The next morning I stood by Dana in the prep room. I kissed him goodbye, but did not say the word.

And he said, "Love Only," as they wheeled him out the back doors. I turned to go out the front. I looked back one last time to see his bed disappear through the sliding door. Ever since the news of the tumour I'd been strong and sane. Yes, I'd been angry but not over the top. I'd been sad but I had stayed away from the blackness of despair. I'd been brave, too, brave enough to sign the papers and take the role of a wife when all I felt like was a desperate child. I'd been graceful enough to let my mother comfort me.

But when I saw my husband disappear, possibly forever, I had nothing left to hold me up. My legs gave out, and I crumpled to the floor.

23

I slept through his surgery. It was a good escape. I woke in time
to join the celebration: Dana was alive, the surgery had been perfect.
He'd have a long road to recovery. But not too long. Two hours after he
came to, Dana was calling for water and pillow adjustments.

"ICU patients don't talk, they groan," a nurse chided on the way back
through the curtain.

Not Dana. He complained loudly about oxygen tubes and a fat head
and the catheter that was placed all wrong. He called the nurses sweetie
and honey and he said damn and shit and hell. He begged me to swab
his dry, stinky mouth, and when I did, he would bite down on the stick
and suck with all his might. The tiny damp sponge could never satisfy
his thirst.

The nurse eventually relented and let me give him ice chips. But she
and the rest of the unit heard him cheering and yelling for more ice
between every mouthful. So she came back in and took the chips away.

"Sorry, I'm not having my neurosurgery patient vomiting on my
watch."

He was mad when she left, but I was thrilled. My Dana was awake
and funny and defiant, drunk with painkillers, but Dana just the same,
and I knew that he would be all right.

It was a rough week, an emotional roller coaster of good days and
very bad days, but one week after surgery Dana walked out of the hospital. I drove him home. He was positive and determined. He kept his
sense of humour even though he was medicated and bald and stapled
in a zig-zag all the way across the top of his head from one ear to the

other. He gained weight. His only complaint was not feeling his scalp or knowing where the top was. But he did not have headaches, not even from smashing his head on the headboard and the cabinets and the frame of the car every time he got in or out of it.

"You have to be positive, Autumn." We were eating in a restaurant, celebrating our first wedding anniversary. "It's the only way to get through stuff like this. It's the reason I'm healing so fast. You gotta laugh. You just gotta laugh."

I did laugh. For joy, for relief, for thanks, for strength to face the next day. I laughed in wonder, too. Dana's recovery was a miracle, but not the only miracle. To that point it was the worst experience of my life. And I had gotten through it without going crazy. At least not wholly crazy. I had put off crazy and fragile for as long as I could. A couple of weeks at least. But it wasn't long before it found me again.

Soon.

Dana was on his feet, getting back to normal. And soon I was on my back, getting back to being me. My obstetrician noticed I was dilating far too early and experiencing irritable little contractions far too often.

"Any stress in your life?"

"Oh, like my husband just had brain surgery two weeks ago?"

"What? Why didn't you say so?"

He admitted me to the pre-term labour unit, where the nurses treated me like a teenage pregnancy. Which, at nineteen, I was.

The first two weeks with an IV pump attached to my left hand made my arms sore. I crocheted an entire baby blanket, flat on my back, while holding my arms and the blanket and the yarn up over my face.

It should have brought good thoughts. But I was consumed by death. I obsessed about suicide, homicide, and infanticide. In meticulous gory detail. This obsession was not like the adolescent's dream of throwing herself dramatically in front of a garbage truck. I was utterly serious. Every waking hour of the day, as I sank ever deeper into a black blanket of flannel, I wanted it. Death.

The obstetrician comes in as he does every morning before breakfast, and today five students follow him. Lucky students doing rounds—

learning the ropes of obstetrics and in my room, incidentally, a bit of psychiatry.

"Good morning, Autumn."

Tell him. Tell him you are going to knife your belly or jump from the roof and tell him about your dream and the demons and the flesh. Tell him. My Girl is on a rant. She wants to take over and tell on me, so they will know and protect me. I don't want their protection. I fight her.

"How are you this morning?" The obstetrician asks.

I can't speak. If I do . . . if I open my mouth, My Girl will tell on me. They'll know I'm nuts. They'll take my baby away from me. Mom will be right about God punishing me for messing around with procreation. *Can't let Mom be right about that.*

"How are you, Autumn?"

I stare at him and hold my mouth closed, and I cry. He stands there looking at me and offers to feel my belly. With a nod I let him, but I am still crying. When he is done, he herds the students into the hall, and I hear him say to the nurse, "Keep an eye on this one—she's very unstable."

And she says, "Right, Autumn Stringam."

Then he says to the med students, "Probably we'll keep her on this ward because they can't do much for her in psych when she's pregnant."

But it is a psych ward in its own way. I'm not allowed to leave my room. They keep me in my bed and they encourage Dana to stay for long visits. But the visits are never long enough, and when he leaves the thoughts take over and I won't tell anyone just how bad it is, until one night I let My Girl make a phone call.

"Come back," she says.

"Hon, is that you?"

"Come here," she says.

"Babe, it's the middle of the night. I have an exam . . ."

"Please come."

He can hear it now, the grunt, the effort, the struggle for control. My Girl is begging, and I am hiding behind her, watching and hearing the voices that tell me how to do the sickest things. The front brain tyrants beat My Girl backward until she is about to drop the phone. She needs both hands to cover the hole that I can feel gaping in my chest. So she can't stay on the phone.

He hears it. "I'm coming."

Dana brings a wheelchair and pulls me out of bed. I put on what I think is a normal face as he wheels me past the nurse's desk into the atrium.

The nurse speaks up: "You're not allowed to take her out of her room, you know."

"Yeah, I know. We'll only be a minute. I need to talk to her."

She gives him a look. *You need to do more than talk to her*.

He sits in front of me and bites the inside of his cheek and cries as I tell him my thoughts. Not all of them, just the most acceptable ones; he couldn't deal with all of them. Just a tiny bit of the workings of my mind.

He does the only thing he knows how to do. He prays over me. He asks God to protect me. He begs God to help me and to keep me safe from all harm or evil. He prays so humbly and so lovingly that God hears his prayers and grants me peace.

In the morning Dana is gone, but I still feel the peace. In the morning I talk to the doctor, and his students listen in. He looks relieved, so they look relieved, and I feel happy. The peace lasts all day. I know it is just one phase of the tide. But I enjoy its presence while I can.

James was worth all I had to endure to get him here. He came out long and skinny and blond. Even before his shoulders were out, the nurses were laughing about his dimples. Dimples. I couldn't get them by boring my fingers into my cheeks, but my son had dimples.

I came home from the hospital to a place filled with new furniture. Dana's gift to me.

Mom and Shawna came to visit for a couple of days to help out with James. We spent most of the time lying on the new furniture, the Hide-A-Bed pulled out, laughing and talking. Mom laughed a lot. She ordered in Chinese food and recited poetry and cried about Dad and his affair of the heart. I thought: This will pass. Just as Dad said, she'll move on. She'll get normal again. She always does.

When they went back to Fort McMurray, I was sad, but spent. Mom's moods were high, going full speed ahead, and mine were in direct contrast, grinding to a dark and painful halt. I felt the low coming, but I had no power to hold it off, let alone turn it away.

I sit on the couch and kiss my baby and smell his sweet head. I want to feel something for this child. I try hard to be normal. I laugh when Dana holds him up and kisses him and talks to him.

Dana, such a great daddy, so in love with his tiny little boy. I want to feel that. I want to feel capable of loving.

I am not a good mom. I struggle for a week or two before a wave, a swollen high tide, sweeps over me. I find a hairdresser to chop my hair off. I dance and pull at my flabby belly and try to squeeze into my teenage clothes. Then, when the high burns out and the tide retreats, I grow sorrowful and sick and weepy as the fungus of darkness grows inside my head.

Dana brings James to me and places him on me to nurse. He rolls me over and moves James to the other side. He changes a diaper and tucks James back into his little bed. I sleep right through it.

Dana is still only a few months out of brain surgery, his hair not yet grown back around the bright red snake of a scar across his scalp. He is tired and drugged on anti-seizure medication. But he is ambitious, trying to get some schooling in while he is on disability. He wants desperately to get out of the box plant job, to get an education and start a career. He wants to do his part for our family. He wants to provide well for his wife and his son. So the nighttime feedings are hard on him. Sometimes he gets angry with me.

"What's the matter with you?" He rocks the bed and shoves my leg to wake me up. "You're supposed to care about him. He needs his mother. Autumn, Autumn, your baby is hungry and he's crying. He needs you."

I shuffle to get his tiny one-month-old body out of the crib. I nurse him in the dark in the living room. My head nods. James falls off my breast. I feel a sudden rage that he won't stay put. I don't want to hurt him, but if he's hungry, he should act like it.

I have to get away from him.

"Dana. Your baby is out on the living room floor."

"What the hell are you talking about?" He is furious. How could I leave an infant—our baby—on the floor in the dark?

I don't know. Don't care. I am flat. I feel nothing. Nothing. I know it isn't right, isn't proper, isn't normal. I just can't make myself feel any different. My heart is dead.

Three months after James is born, I know the truth about Dana. He is plotting my death, he and his gang. The plan is for him to leave the apartment and pretend to lock the door so I will stay in bed and feel safe. Then his craven killers will walk right in and do their dirty work.

He leaves for school. I lie in bed and listen as he closes the apartment door. *Shhhh-bang. Click.* The door locks. *Rattle-click.* There! He's done it! He's unlocked it for the killers. I freeze under the covers for an hour, sometimes two. Until James wakes up screaming. Then I have no choice but to go and get him. But first . . .

I check the lock. Every day it is locked. Then I know for sure. It's tomorrow that they will do the deed.

By lunchtime I see I am fat. I need to exercise. By then Dana is the smartest man on earth. Going to school. I am so proud of him.

By suppertime I am in love with him. I become the best cook this side of the border. At bedtime I am whiny and exhausted and too quiet. And Dana is the best daddy little boy James could ever want.

In the morning he sneaks out and leaves the door unlocked for his gang. And one day they come for me.

Lying cold and stiff and fearful and waiting, I hear the door open. I hear footsteps in the hall. I leap from my bed. I leap onto my killer in the hall. I beat on him. I thrash. I scream. I cry. *Don't kill me, don't kill me. Please don't kill me.*

But no. He will not show me any mercy. He picks me up and hauls me kicking and screaming into the bedroom. He tosses me on my bed.

Go ahead and kill me. I don't care any more. Go on and kill me.

His smile melts. He sees that this is no charade.

"I was just coming back for my books, hon."

And now he knows for certain. It's all out there. I'm all out there, my fraud exposed. "You're sick." As simple as that other on-the-mark diagnosis from not so long ago: It's a brain tumour.

And just as serious. He makes an appointment for me to see a doctor.

I was diagnosed with postpartum depression. My body was weak, and my vision was blurred off and on, and my legs were dragging sometimes, literally dragging, so the doctor tested for multiple sclerosis. Inconclusive—just like everything else in my life. He put me on Prozac.

The Prozac felt good for the first two weeks, but then the agitation set in.

Week three I was angry.

Week four I was flirty. I had my hair chopped even closer to my skull.

Week five I started moving the family to a new apartment and scrubbing everything in sight and threatening to hit James if he didn't shut up.

Week six I was brutal, delusional, manic, scary. And as Dana was driving me to the doctor, I began flapping.

Flapping. He hasn't seen that one before. I am whipping my hands and arms, hard and fast in front of my face, pounding my face, scratching my face. He holds my seat belt closed with one hand and drives with the other as I scream and try to open the door on the freeway to throw myself out into the traffic. He can't do it. He has to drive off the freeway into a neighbourhood.

There he lets me out. "If that's really what you want." He pulls to the curb and undoes my seat belt. "Go."

Flapping, I fly from the car. I flap and bounce in the shade on the sidewalk. I have to get away. He follows me slowly with the car and watches me knocking my head around and rattling my knees and jumping and talking to myself.

He comes out of the car and holds me. I want him to hold me. But I still can't stop flapping my hands. So he puts me back in the car and drives me to the doctor's office.

The frenzied, raging, angry part is over. I am crying. I beg the doctor to make it stop. My legs shake; my arms burn. My face stings.

"Oh, Autumn, I didn't know you were bipolar," the doctor says. "I thought we were dealing with a simple postpartum depression."

"Please make this stop."

I see Dana standing in the corner of the office with his hands deep in his pockets. He is chewing the inside of his cheek.

The doctor goes out and comes back with a needle full of sleep. He sticks it in my bum, and I feel the warmth of it in just seconds.

I'm so-o-o sleepy. He asks me a question.

Wha-a-a-ah?

"Who else in your family is a manic depressive?"

Oh, now I understand. Not only the question. And not only the answer. But also my entire life. *Who else indeed?*

24

Mom. I thought I knew her, now that I knew the monster possessing me had possessed her first. I told her I'd found relief. I was off Prozac and onto lithium and Paxil and an occasional tranquilizer. I wanted her to know she could get help.

I went into the closet in the back room of our basement apartment and dragged the phone in, trailing the cord under the door. I called her from a tight space where I could see all the boundaries of my world, a safe place. I told her I was feeling different, even better—but Mom, back at the centre of the universe, wasn't listening.

She went on about how she was born into the wrong family, how she was supposed to have been born as a sister to her friend Cory. He was in nearly every conversation now, and I was sick of it.

"Mom, you aren't making sense."

"You can't see it? We were meant to be. We're soulmates."

"Are you having an affair?"

"What? Don't be sick. You know I'd never . . . you know I would never commit adultery. It's not like that. It's just that Cory understands me. He's my spirit brother."

"Mom, why don't you just leave Cory out of your life?"

"Don't tell me how to live, you little druggie."

"What?"

"You're a little lithium head. A druggie. And fat, too."

"Mom, stop."

She laughed and hung up. She went away. She called back later and kept calling, but she had left our reality and never came back. She obsessed about Cory. Obsessed about Dad. She was going to do great things. She started taking singing lessons and launched another home business. She took to country music. Her songs changed, her voice changed. She talked about the spiritual connection between Cory's family and ours, the mistake in the universe that had kept them apart for so many years.

Then, one day, she told me that Cory was moving to southern Alberta with his family. *Good*, I thought. Maybe she'd find something else to talk about, maybe get some help.

A short time later she started a conversation with, "So I started packing today."

"What?"

"Yeah, I told your father that we're moving to Cardston. I'm going to go find us a house."

She was moving to stay near Cory? "What about Dad's company? There's no property management work in Cardston."

"He'll sell it."

"Can he support the family with a new business?"

"Don't care. I'm going, and no one is stopping me. I told him I'm going, and he can come if he wants to."

"Mom . . ."

"Okay, well, I'm busy. See ya." *Click.*

She packed up the home in Fort McMurray, and, of course, Dad went with her to Cardston. Of course. He tried to keep the family together and lost everything else. They bought a tiny two-storey stone house with a spiral staircase, on a corner lot lined with century-old trees. Her dream house—with brown shag to boot. Her dream, but Dad's failure. He lost his company, the airplane, the respect he'd earned in years of building a business. The house in Fort McMurray didn't sell, so the bank repossessed it. When the savings were gone and the investments had dried up, he lost his last remaining shred of dignity. He went on the road to sell dog food in a multi-level marketing company. Meanwhile, the Stephan kids ran wild in a tiny town where everyone knows your name.

Dad's income didn't cover the new mortgage and the food and

clothes for the eight children at home. The tax bill for the previous year came in, but the money was gone. The savings were spent, and Dad was scrambling for new work that would let him stay close to home. Mom took a job as a teacher's aide, but she lost it her first day.

Revenue Canada started calling, demanding payment. Water from a stone, he told them, no money to pay. They ate beans and oatmeal and wheat, boiled and fried, or popped dry if there was no butter or oil. Revenue Canada tried to garnishee Dad's meagre income. Dad couldn't pay, but they didn't believe him.

It was all falling apart. Mom, angry and illogical, stormed the community with accusations and innuendo about Dad. And worse, there were rumours about Mom and Cory meeting at the public library, reciting poetry to each other. There was more than talk; there was action. The poetic pair were scheming and dreaming. They came up with plans for a partnership, a recording business complete with a studio. Mom fed the rumour mill, confiding in her aunts and cousins and neighbours, daughters, clergymen, and doctors.

Dad, as usual, was desperate to keep it all together. Desperate to defend her, to shield her, to keep up the act. "It's okay," he'd say. "Everything is normal here. She'll come out of it, and things will get normal again—she always does, and they always do."

He was desperate and desolate and determined. But it wasn't working any more. The kids went hungry, and Mom went wild. Dad was used up, drowning in denial. Then, just when it seemed things could not get worse, they did.

Thanksgiving. A time for family and friends and good food and good times. I don't know what I was thinking. I knew before we went that the gathering would go bad. We drove to Cardston. It was the first time I had been in her new house, her dream house. As Dana turned the corner into the driveway, I thought we had the wrong place. The woman at the door had long pale-blonde hair and was thinner than Mom.

"Is that your mom?"

"Uh . . ." *I hope not.* "I think so."

Some of the kids ran up behind her. We recognized them. So it was Mom. I was glad to see them and even her. I missed home. I missed my family. And I saw at first glance why it was the dream house. She had the shag carpeting again.

Saturday I awoke to the thump of music from the stereo. I pried open an eye to see that it was barely five o'clock. I slumped out of bed and cracked open the guest room door to find all of the lights on. I saw Mom dressed in tight blue jeans and one of my sweaters from high school. She was dancing as she vacuumed the long brown strands of shag. She waved to me and smiled. *Just another day in the neighbourhood.*

We didn't last twenty-four hours. Mom slapped little Jeremy for not having socks on and left welts on his cheeks. I was disgusted. To get even, I called her the worst name possible: Grandma.

She freaked. "I'm too young for that crap. Don't you lump me in with Old Lady Stringam."

"Age has nothing to do with it. I'm your daughter, and this is my son. That makes you a grandmother."

"I wish you were never born," she said. I don't know how she meant it exactly. *If you weren't born, I wouldn't have to face being a grandma?* Or, *I hate your guts?* Either way, it left a welt of a different kind, on my heart.

Dana loaded the car, I put James in, and we drove away. I'd never felt so low.

25

We skipped Christmas with Mom and Dad. Dana wanted to build memories for James that did not include my fighting with Mom and crying all the way home.

But we could not skip Angela's missionary farewell. It was the second week of January 1994. Angela was to go to a training centre to learn Dutch. Then she'd be off to Belgium for eighteen months. The farewell should have been about Angela. But, as usual, it was all about Debora. Her hair was now black, and she was thinner than ever before. She was more glazed, dark, and sarcastic than I'd ever seen her.

Mom gave a talk in church that Sunday at Angela's farewell. I'd never seen her so vicious outside the house. I had never thought she would humiliate her entire family from the pulpit.

She hinted at her sorrows for being married to a man like *him*. She talked of overcoming adversity in spite of *him*.

She was attacking Dad in a farewell for her daughter? Furious and disgusted, I stopped listening. And soon enough I became angry with Dad instead of her. Why didn't he get a spine? Stand up for himself! Dana would never take such criticism from me; why is he taking it from her?

She didn't talk about Angie leaving. She talked about her own leaving. I felt sick to my stomach. She was telling the world that she was leaving. Leaving Dad.

Later we choked down a dinner and posed for a family picture. It had been four years since our last photo as a whole family, she said and insisted. We gathered on and around the couch in the front parlour. Mom, Dad, and all the rest of us—nine children, and Dana and James.

Sometimes I still look at this photo to remember what it is I want to forget. At first glance it looks as if the whole family is there. On second glance I can see Mom's body, a shell without a soul. She is glazed and dark in the eyes. Her smile is frozen, grim. The rest of us are grim, too, tolerating the moment that she insists on having with us. *We are grim because of her awful behaviour.*

She is grim because she knows.

This is no Kodak moment.

This is goodbye.

Two weeks later I turn twenty-one and Mom doesn't call. It's Friday and I cry all night over Mom and the phone call she didn't make today. Dana says I don't need that family any more—we'll make our own.

At least Angela will have a birthday recognition. I sent a package to her in the mission training centre; her twenty-second birthday will be on Monday. But when Monday comes I am not at home, and Angela is not celebrating her birthday.

Mom is dead, and I am at her side with Dad.

In the mortuary.

She has killed herself while Dad was far away, on a business trip to Utah. She drove the family van to Woolford Provincial Park, attached a hose to the exhaust pipe, and filled the cab with deadly gas. Dana and I drove all through the night arriving in Cardston a few hours before Dad drove up to find all of his children and half of mom's family mourning in the living room of Mom's dream house.

On Monday night I start making the phone calls.

"Hello, Uncle Bruce, are you sitting down?"

Dad sits and listens to me calling and reporting the news of Mom's death. "No, he can't come to the phone right now. Can you come to the funeral?"

I hang up and Dad is staring into space, slumped on the desk. "Are you okay?"

"No."

"Do you want me to keep calling?"

Dad covers his mouth with his arm while the tears roll onto his sleeve. I can't look at him. I pick up the receiver and dial the next number.

"Hello, Doug? Are you sitting down?"

On Tuesday morning I wake before sunrise to the sound of my dad pacing in the kitchen, tromping about with his shoes on. His pace is erratic, shuffling on the dirty floor as he turns to double back in the other direction. I slip out from under Dana's arm. Dana likes the window open, and the January wind whistles its way in. The carpet is iced under my feet. I feel pangs of guilt as I pull my sweater over my head, the static lifting my short hair and sticking it to my forehead and earlobes. I was sleeping while he was pacing. I should have been there for him when he came downstairs.

The wind outside the open window has created a vacuum in the room, so the door sucks and snaps as I pull it open. Dad hears and comes quickly around the corner to greet me. His face is blocked partly by the tightly twisted spiral staircase that creaks and rattles between us.

"Hi," he says.

"Hi." My throat is sore, and my voice cracks on the word.

I follow him into the kitchen. We chat about food and cold rooms and drafty windows. The house is quiet. Most of the crying aunts and friends have found their way to other places to sleep for the night.

Our voices carry up the carpeted spiral to my sisters, Angela and Sunni, who creak down the stairs one after the other.

"Angie," I say. "You made it back."

"Yeah, Sunni and Joe picked me up in Calgary last night. I got on the first flight after they told me."

Dad doesn't remember it was Angela's birthday yesterday. Her birthday may never have a place in his memory again. Not after what Mom has done. *On the eve of her eldest daughter's birthday?*

I've drifted from the conversation. I try to catch up to the instructions Dad is giving Angie and Sunni.

"I'm so sorry," he says. "She always said that she would only want me to do it, but I can't. I just can't . . ." His voice cracks. He rubs his unshaven jowl and nose, turning away from us.

We know what we must do. There's a viewing tonight and the funeral tomorrow. Angela, Sunni, and I need to dress Mom's body for burial.

We dig through the pile in the entryway to find our boots and coats among the heap of shoes and outdoor wear. We trudge through the snowbanks to reach my car.

"What should we do first?" Sunni asks.

"Let's go see when the clothing store opens and then go down and get Marie," Angela says. "She's a hairdresser. She wants to help. We should let her."

We get to the clothing store just as it opens and file inside to the customer service desk. None of us has dressed a dead body before. We ask for a bit of help picking out the clothes.

The woman at the desk nods. She knows. She walks us to the back, a place the public does not see. She unveils a huge assortment of gowns and other burial fashions.

"What size is she, Angie?" I finger my way through a rack of white satin and lace.

"Pretty close to yours," she says. "These are pretty baggy anyway, so we just need to worry about the fit in the shoulders."

My size. She had always made such a big deal about my being thin. Then when I got fat with James and stayed that way with lithium, she tried to get smaller.

"Before I die, I'll be skinnier than you," she told me once. You win, Deb. You win again.

We choose a lovely white ankle-length gown adorned with lace and satin. We purchase a slip, stockings, slippers, and all of the trimmings that Mom would have chosen for herself. None of us have money to spare, but none of us mention it. Together we seem strong.

I feel strong enough to say, "Let's not get Marie yet. We can do this. Mom wanted family to do it."

"Okay. We won't get her yet."

We go through the heavy mortuary doors, feeling strong together. *We'll do it for Dad. We'll do it for Mom.*

Mom is at the far end of the room. An ironing board, a spray bottle, and a table stand by, ready for us to put a final press on her clothes. I march up to Mom's side. I empty the bag on the table and begin to sort the clothes in the order they will be placed on her body. Then I look for my sisters. Sunni is looking in the empty casket.

"Pretty, isn't it?" I stroke the white satin lining and run my fingers over the tapestry flowers and pewter handles that adorn her vault.

"Who picked it out?"

"Dad and I. We thought this sort of suited her."

"Yeah."

We hear a moan. Angela. Sunni and I turn to see her seeing Mom for the first time this way. Because suicide from carbon dioxide turns the skin a bluish-grey, someone has painted her face and hands—the parts that will show—with a lurid orangey makeup. Angela strokes Mom's hair. She cries, and we join her, three sisters, so different, but so much in common, daughters of a mother who killed herself. I hold Mom's feet. Angela is at her head and Sunni is at her elbow. We cry and howl over Mom's body until the wails and heaves and sobs blend together and we are one voice.

I can't take it. I'm at my limit. I know I will bolt from here.

It's okay. I feel her come to me . . . Thank you, thank you. I relinquish control to My Girl.

"Okay," she says to my sisters, "let's get this done."

We work for hours. Dad comes in to check on us and so does a tall grey man. We don't want the mortician there, and Dad finds excuses to whisk him right back out the doors.

At the end of the day I am alone again with Mom. Final details, primping. I welcome the solitude, and I'm just not ready to leave. Not yet.

I run my hand over the casket and breathe deep, fingering the pewter handles and the fine satin edging. This one *is* special. The tapestry is all floral with pinks and blues and muted indigo. The blue-green leaves are like the ones she painted in our living room in Fort McMurray. I remember her then, the day she painted that, a good memory. I let it wash over me, bringing a smile and a chuckle. Until . . .

"Oh, Mom, your hands have curled up again." I am talking out loud. "I've spread your hands out at least ten times today. Why do they keep going back?"

I hold her hands, untangling the fingers that have recurled around each other. They are as stiff and cold as damp clay. I admire again the length of her slender fingers and run the tips of my fingers, with their bitten-down nails, over the soft rounded bitten-down tips of hers. I think of how her hands were peacekeepers and warmongers, how they were kind and harsh and swift and gentle. They embodied all that she was to me. These hands that nursed her babies and created beautiful artistry, the same hands that bloodied my nose and pointed in mockery . . . they are beautiful to me now. I rub and rub until the warmth of my living palms relaxes the joints of her fingers and releases the bend of her wrist.

Gently, I position her hands on her chest, folding them together, as if she were in solemn prayer. Or an angel.

26

Dad is numb. And angry. He stands at the viewing with his hands tight and his jaw clenched. He is keeping everything inside and doing his best to seem normal. There are people coming and going that I have not seen in years. People who lost touch with our family have come to share our pain. Or maybe just to gawk.

After most of the others have gone, I shuffle up next to Dad to touch his arm. He is looking at her. I need to touch him, to let him know that there is no blame on him. *And none on me, right, Dad? You don't blame me either. Right, Dad?*

"She was possessed." He is looking into her pretty box.

"What?"

"It's not her fault. She didn't do this. She was possessed." His jaw is set. He's firm about this. It's not her fault.

He is right, I suppose. "She was sick," I say.

Dad shakes his head, he doesn't understand *sick*, not this kind of sick. He needs someone to blame, and the devil is a proper scapegoat.

"She never could have done this on her own." Back into denial; he'll never, never, never give up on her.

"I know, Dad, it wasn't her. She didn't choose this." I can say the words for his sake, although I don't have the same conviction.

"I saw it, you know. The whole thing." He shudders.

No, he didn't. He wasn't there. On Sunday afternoon he was still in Utah, selling dog food. He drove all night to get to us, to get back to her. Unless . . .

"How, Dad?" I ask. "How did you see it?"

Dad's eyes fill with tears as he leans forward a little to brace himself on the coffin. He speaks in a whisper.

"I was driving back from Utah, and I knew she was gone. All of a sudden she was with me in the car." He pauses and leans forward and whispers, "Her perfume, so close to me. Like when we used to drive around and hold hands, like last week before I left for the trip, like when you were kids on the acreage. I saw our life, and her death. She told me everything, and I saw it all—all of it. And she was sorry, and then she was gone. She was just gone."

"Oh, Dad."

He shoves his hands in his pockets and pulls out a napkin to wipe his face and eyes. "At least she came to say goodbye."

Normal people don't understand the eyes, the heart, the mind of a suicide. It doesn't make sense to people like Dad and Angela. It would never make sense to Dana. But it makes sense to me. When my eyes go blank, I'll be desperate for relief, too. I'll do anything to escape the torment. Anything. I can't blame her for that. I can't blame her for escaping, and now I know that sooner or later I'll escape, too.

But not today. And not tomorrow. Tomorrow we have the funeral.

Tomorrow comes, and we start the routine again. Waking and eating. Dressing the children, dressing ourselves. We dread this day, the funeral. Most of all we dread the people. But we do it anyway, for Mom. Another day of the formalities of grieving.

I am so tired. I know now why they drag out the ceremony of death. The vigils and praying and viewings and funeral and burial and meals and condolences and more. It's so you'll be so exhausted that you won't have the strength to be angry. So exhausted that you won't talk. So exhausted that when you see your Uncle Gordy and his daughters at the funeral, you won't remember why you hate him. So exhausted you won't remember to tremble for his daughters.

So very exhausted that when they lower the pretty box into the frozen ground, you won't protest. Instead you'll say: Good riddance. Finally, it's over. Now can I please get some sleep?

We stand for an hour, lined up straight like a scene from *The Sound of Music*. The father in his suit, his children at attention, spiffed up and smelling clean. But we are not happy, we are not singing. And no one wants to look at us. We form an aisle for the grievers and the gawkers to pass through. A husband and nine children on one side: Angela, Autumn, Sunni, Daniel, Bradford, Joseph, David, Jeremy, and Celeste. Evidence that she lived.

And on the other side Mom's dead body laid out, proof that she died. Which was more pleasant to look at? The motherless children, the abandoned husband? Or the cold woman, tight-fisted, her skin stained orange with mortician's makeup?

People kiss us and hug us and look at Mom's body and grimace. They hug us again and some of them weep so hard we have to hold them up and comfort them. *Why is that our job when we can barely stand ourselves?*

When we push the coffin into the chapel, I wail out loud, a sudden burst of emotion that escapes before I can snatch it back. People are staring. People know me. *Autumn. Again.*

They're right to be fearful. I've cycled from yesterday's understanding into anger again, an anger I can barely control. I gather myself on the bench and try to vent it silently before it's time for me to say the opening prayer. But there just isn't enough time to swing back to tranquility.

I feel a flame-up as I get to my feet. At the pulpit, I say aloud what nobody else would even whisper. "Heavenly Father, we are gathered here together in grief and ask Thee to bless us as we mourn the suicide of Debbie Stephan . . ."

The congregation lets out an audible gasp at the word. What did they expect? We mourn the *passing*? We mourn the *untimely death*? There is no kind way to put it. My mother killed herself. It wasn't quick or accidental. No impassioned slip of the knife or tug on the trigger. It was an intentional, deliberate, premeditated, and well-planned murder of herself. *It was suicide, people, suicide.*

In a way, it's funny. Here is Autumn—volatile, angry lunatic that she is—standing in front of the congregation with the weapon of the public address system at hand. Just like Mom at Angie's mission farewell. And nobody but Autumn can control Autumn now. Whose great idea was this, anyhow?

Dad's. It was Dad's idea. So I have to control my mouth for him. I'll do it for Dad.

Inside, though, I rage at Mom for paying double on her life insurance. *Did you know that, people?* That she said her goodbyes in letters written months in advance? That she had one last family photo taken, knowing all the while it would be the very last? That she waited until Dad was too far away to save her from herself? Too far away to get home before all of the children found out she'd disappeared? Too far away even to get home before her body was discovered? I want to say it to their pious faces. Tell them outright in the middle of their solemn ceremony. Shock them with the awful reality.

Did you know that she lied to him over the phone the morning that she ditched us, acting normal, talking about a winter storm in the forecast? That all the while she was in the middle of packing up her van with the poetry and the pillows and the vacuum cleaner hose, telling him, "Oh, yeah, everything is fine . . . Kids, yeah, they're good. They miss you . . . When do you think you'll start back?" Knowing full well it would be later that day, long after she had vanished. Knowing he would get the call: *Dad, Mom is gone . . . I don't know, just gone. We can't find her, Dad, we can't find her.* Knowing he would start driving back right away.

I am furious that she played us like a board game. When all the pieces lined up, it was her final sick victory. She fooled him, tricked us, and came out the winner in a game of strategy where only she knew the rules. We didn't know the rules and we never saw it coming. *Ha. Ha. See? I win again. See? See?*

I choke on my rage, but I choke it back, too.

Yes, I am Autumn and crazy. But not so crazy or so much like my mother that I will shame my dad at a time like this. Or maybe I simply will not afford everyone the gossip. I will not share the awful, shameful details of my crazy mother's death. I stick to my prayer. And after, when I sit down again, I feel the congregation, including my family and even the church building itself, breathe a collective sigh of relief.

27

We buried Mom on a hill overlooking the town. The interment should have been sad, peaceful, spiritual. But I was robbed of these feelings by the anger.

Dana and I drove out to the graveyard in our own car. I needed to breathe before taking on the family and the church and the neighbours again. I needed to cry out loud and only with Dana. I needed to speak my mind, bare my soul, but I couldn't. It was only a five-minute drive to the grave, barely long enough to catch my breath and cry a little and worry about my failing legs.

Others stood at the graveside, but I sat. Front row and centre, next to little CC. Dana took care of his pallbearer duties and then came to stand behind me. He held my shoulder, but I slumped away from him, slouching in the chair and holding my knees for support.

I was drowning in the moment, suddenly very aware of this scene: my mother in a coffin propped over a deep hole; mounds of dirt disguised with a tarp; the flowers, the faces. Each face with its own story of Deb, each face a slice of history within her lifetime. Each with its own tale of laughter, anger, love, or pain. Each face looking to the next face for comfort, for relief, for an absolution of guilt.

They will find no comfort in my face. I dare you to tell the truth about what you knew. What you saw, what you did to kill her, or what you didn't do to save her. I dare you. I scan the faces with my daring bloodshot stare.

I see Dad at the head of the grave, clutching his white leather-bound scriptures to his chest, preparing to give the dedicatory prayer.

I see Angela and Sunni, tired and weeping and leaning against their boyfriends for support.

I hear voices. The sound of people whispering and mourning. Explanations and introductions and gossip. I want to tell them to shut up, to have respect, to forget what they think they know and to know only that she was not at all what she became or seemed to become. They didn't know her heart. They only knew her moods.

In truth, they didn't know her at all. I knew her. Yes, before she was dead, she was maniacal, and before the mania, obsessed. Before the obsession she was depressed, and before that tired. But before all of these things, she was my mother, and I loved her.

Dad is talking now. His prayer is soft and pleading, and I don't want to hear it. I have to go. The crowd is behind me. Up is the only way out. I pull up and away into the scenery, into the wind. I will find a memory to keep of this day, and it won't be the faces surrounding Mom. My Girl will keep those images, those questions. My memory will be only of the place where we left Mom. I will remember this place as beautiful.

I see the graveyard on this hill set in the middle of farms and ranches, framed by majestic evergreens, planted by those long dead. The trees, although well rooted and staked to lean into the west wind, have been forced over the years of gale-force storms to bow to the east. Here the wind is a sea, heavy and full and consistent. Pressing and whipping, clean and crisp and warm and always there in summer, neverending in winter. The tide rolls from the west, the chinook wind rolls off the face of Chief Mountain, sacred to the Blood, the Blackfoot, and the Peigan, the people of the Blackfoot Nation. The Chief gives life and provides warmth as he breathes the chinook, melting the snow and exposing the tawny fields for the grazers. He keeps a food source readily available for the hunters.

There are no flowers on the graves. Every other day they tumble and careen before the riptides of wind, flying from the vases, leaping over tombstones to collect in a tangle against the east fence line. But today is different, rare. Today the great and ever-present sea of wind lies calm, the tides at rest, subdued by the sound of Dad's prayer, silent in respect for our tears, none more bitter than mine.

Because I know what happened now. Because she speaks to my heart. Because she tells me she is sorry now that she killed herself. Because she knows she made a mistake and is willing to admit it.

That's supposed to make me forgive her, and I might well forgive her, in time. But not today.

28

When you die, your privacy dies with you. Eventually, someone will rifle through your purse, your bathroom cabinet, your pockets. Someone will discover your journal and your secret feelings, all of your angriest and silliest and most lustful thoughts on paper. Someone will notice the stains in the underarms of your T-shirts, the hole in your worn-out underwear, the stash of candy in your bottom dresser drawer, the birthday gift that you shoved to the very back of your closet in the box marked "Yard Sale." Eventually, all your secrets are told, all of you discovered and exposed. Perhaps this is the scariest part about dying. The living go on to know you better than you might have wanted. When you die, their discoveries will lift you on a pedestal or diminish your legacy.

Dad didn't want to live without Mom, and he didn't want Mom to be discovered and exposed and diminished. But he could no longer protect her.

Her suicide note, catalogued by the police along with all of the other evidence seized from the van, said so much. It had been written weeks before, when Revenue Canada had attempted to take Dad's wages from his bank account, but there was no money to take. The family was destitute. She told Dad he was a damn good man; she told him she was sorry. She asked him to use the money from her life insurance to pay off the taxman, so Revenue Canada would stop harassing the family. She asked Dad to pay her debts and use the rest to make ends meet for the seven children who were still at home.

So he did. He took the insurance money and wrote a cheque. He sent me to pay the debt. I cried all the way to the tax office. When I got in, I told the cashier that they had harassed my mother to death and I hoped the money was worth it to them.

Dad was sure Mom was with him: in the house, in the car, in his mind and heart. She was with him, and he wanted to spare her all embarrassment. He wanted to preserve her in the everyday. So he left things as she left them. For months her perfume and toothbrush lay on the bathroom counter. Her shoes stood in a careful row in front of the closet. Her bra and underwear and a fresh towel lay folded on the shelf where she had left them. The room held its breath, waiting for her as if she were simply taking an extra-long shower.

He left her purse and all of her personal things untouched until Celeste, now six years old, got sick.

He calls me in the middle of the afternoon. It is the third time today.

"Autumn, CC is sick, and—"

"Do you need me to come down? I can be there—"

"No. That's not why I'm calling. I had to go into Deb's purse. I wasn't snooping. I just needed to get the Alberta health care cards."

"Well, that's okay." He's worried about snooping. I love him so.

"No, it isn't. Did you know that she was on Prozac?"

"What?"

"I found a bottle, a new prescription. She filled it just a few weeks before she . . ."

"What?" And she called me a druggie?

"I talked to the doctor, and he told me she had been treated for bipolar. Like you. She didn't tell me, Autumn. She didn't tell me that she was taking drugs."

"Wow, Dad, both Mom and me?" In truth I'm not all that stunned by the news she was bipolar. It's been clear to me for a long time. What stuns me is that Dad has kept himself so blind to it all this time.

"And Grandpa, too, Autumn. He had it, too. He killed himself."

I am shocked into silence.

"You didn't know that?"

"No, Dad. When we were little, Mom used to say that he ate too much salt and died. When I was older, she called it a system failure. She said it took him three days to die. His kidneys. And liver. And then his heart . . . *Oh-h-h*." I see now.

"Prescription drug overdose." Dad is nearly reverent with the words. He knows I have drugs, lots and lots of them, in bottles stacked on top of my fridge.

The Prozac bottle was a revelation and a relief to me. It meant that all of her name-calling and cruelty about my own diagnosis and acceptance of treatment was an act. She had recognized the illness in herself. She had sought help. What went wrong? She didn't have enough Prozac in her system? That had to be it. Too little, too late. Never mind what the drug did to me. She was not me. It might have worked for her. She'd taken too long to get help, too long to listen to her doctor.

Not me. I could do better than Mom. I vowed to be a most loyal psychiatric patient. Mom simply didn't understand where to put her trust. She should have trusted Dad. She should have trusted her doctor. She should have taken more drugs.

I trust my physician. I trust in his wisdom. He will care for me, watch over and protect me. I take my drugs and trust them.

It will never end for me as it did for Mom.

Except. I do so hate the drugged feeling, the flatness of emotions, the thickness of my body, the density of my mood. I hate the agitation of the anti-depressant. I fear the darkness of my anti-psychotic meds. I detest the weight gain. I cry at the joint pain. I long for my memory.

More and more, as my memory fails me, I live in an unending stupor. A word on the tip of my tongue that can never be spoken, a constant case of *Dang it, what was I going to tell you? It slipped my mind.* Those drugs. Not even My Girl can keep my memory when I'm crashed on the drugs.

Still. I want to live. *Don't I?* I can spend my life avoiding death. *Can't I?* I won't end up like her, after all. *Will I?*

29

In May Dad went back to Fort McMurray for a visit. He borrowed a van because he could never drive his own van again, the one she had used to kill herself. There he spent time with Barb, Mom's friend. Barb loved Mom and shared Dad's grief.

And then . . .

Dad told me he and Barb were going to get married in the summer and asked if I could please clean out Mom's closet. It was time to put away her things, box up her shoes, and empty her drawers. Throw away her toothbrush and deodorant stick, divide up her keepsakes among the children.

"You're going to get married?"

"Yes."

After only six months? "Dad. So soon?"

"Yes."

So. I cleaned out the closet. And I did it angrily. I snatched clothes from hangers, kicking the fallen pieces into a heap. I ripped out the contents of drawers and punched them down into boxes. I screamed at the shoes, hissed at the toothbrush. I pinched my nose and pursed my lips and tried hard not to smell her in the closet. I cursed the way she permeated the dresses, blue jeans, sweaters, and nightgowns. Each piece was bathed in her. The sweet perfumed scent, mixed with Tide laundry detergent, hair conditioner, and the essence of her skin, filled my mind with music and memories and misery. I tried to stay angry, to rile myself to new heights of rage, but the smell of her broke me. I melted into a heap, slumping over in a puddle of tears on the closet floor. *How could she?*

And now, how could he?

Dad and Barb married in August. I spent my fourth wedding anniversary making my dad's wedding cake. Barb and her six-year-old daughter, Jennifer, moved into the Cardston home. It hurt to see my dad take another wife. The adult part of me could see why it was necessary. The rest of me hated it. I wasn't over Mom yet; heck, some of the boys still hadn't shed real tears over her. No one was over Mom. Not even Dad. Still, he needed a wife. For himself and for his family.

Compared to Barb's situation, I had no reason to complain. She took on the remnants of Debbie's messy life—*and willingly*. Sunni, Daniel, Brad, Joe, David, Jeremy, and Celeste were still at home. Barb's marriage was a mix of two families, with four teenagers and a dash of suicide. Then, to top it off, she became pregnant.

Dad started a new life without ever leaving his old one or his grief. Losing Mom was not the same as divorcing her. He never stopped loving her.

Barb was good to Dad. She gave him space. She let him keep the old family pictures on the wall. She stood by her man, a man obsessed with trying to understand his first wife's death. What right did I have to act as if I were the injured party?

Besides, Dana and I had our own worries and struggles. Viral meningitis put Dana in the hospital for a week, and I was recovering from breaking my back in a car accident. Broken back, broken mind, broken family. Maybe a baby could fix things.

James had turned two and I was baby-hungry. I talked to my doctor even before I talked to Dana. I insisted that I was well enough. He said I could try it. Dana begged me not to. I did it anyway.

I went off my drugs to prepare my body for a pregnancy. Three days into my cleansing I went over: a full-blown psychotic episode complete with voices, visions, flaps and slaps, and punches.

I stayed over. One year and four drugs later, I was still gone.

I was far from where I had started, where I had been somewhat stable. And as much as I wanted it, I could not claw my way back up the cavern wall to stability; I could not do it. The doctor tried new drugs, different cocktails, different sedatives, but my cycle had changed from the long swings of a grandfatherly pendulum to that of a twisted dual-pendulum four-handed clock, the likes of which even Alice in Wonderland had never seen.

I lost myself in the rhythm and the madness.

The doctor told me to get my tubes tied. The newest drug combination would be a disaster for a baby. The possibility of getting normal *and* having a family was out of the question. I could never come off the drugs, never hope for another child. Never again.

"Accept it, Autumn, and then live your life. You are lucky to still have your husband and your son. Give me two years, and we'll find a treatment that works for you."

I listened, but I couldn't bring myself to have the surgery. My Girl wouldn't let me.

When I wasn't writing my illness in poetry and prose, I was singing it to James. I became the queen of impromptu verses. James didn't get it, but Dana did. He heard the messages hidden in the tunes, and he didn't like them.

Row, row, row, your boat, gently down the stream,
till Autumn kicks a hole in it and then you'll hear her scream.
I row and row and row and row, but I don't have an oar
and so sometimes I think that life is really quite a chore.

A chore, so let me out, and I will go and you'll be free.
For happiness will never come when Dana's stuck with me.

"Stop it, Autumn."

"Stop what?"

"The death wish."

"I can't live in this head. You don't understand. I can't last."

"You can't do what your mom did. You can't do that to James." There it was. His greatest fear. And Dad's. And mine.

"I won't." *I guess.*

"Promise me."

I couldn't. So I did the next best thing.

30

I want to be here. I really do. It's the safest place. It really is.
You'll see, my sweet, sweet Dana. He sits on the edge of my bed and
watches me change into the blue cotton backless gown. He knows I
can't deal with this. So he holds another gown for me. This one I'll wear
backward. I have to be covered both ways. This'll be just fine, my sweet,
just fine. You'll see.

I have this nice bed. See? See how I can get on and off the bed? And
this lovely bathroom. Oh, and I have a view of the roof from my sealed,
locked, stupid, unopenable window. *See? See?*

He sits still. I prowl. He cries. I don't.

"I can't do it," he says.

Do what, my sweet?

"I can't leave you here."

I hold up my wrist. *See?* I already have on the printed bracelet. It's
colour-coded, my bracelet of many colours. The many colours mean I
can't leave.

I'm glad, my sweet. Glad that I can't leave, you see? And that I'm
here in this lovely, lovely room. I am relieved, you see? Grateful, you
see? You think it's easy getting into a psych ward?

Don't you see?

No, of course you don't.

You'd have to hear the voices, see the demons in the mirrors. You'd
have to shower with your clothes on. You'd have to clutch them to you
as the water runs so your undershirt won't fall off your shoulders, your

panties won't slip off in the shower. You can't let them slip. Oops, no, no, no slipping.

You'd have to pretend not to hear when the floating faces, those sketchy-looking creatures with the pointed foreheads and the pointed chins, come calling. But you don't hear them, and you don't notice when they are laughing at you, darting low to look into your eyes, rising above you to find your weakest parts.

You don't know how to behave when they come calling, my sweet.

When they say these things, you must close your eyes and sing a song, sing it louder than their voices and make it a religious tune from Sunday school, one with fervour and high-pitched notes to drown them out. Just don't open your eyes, and when they are angry because you won't, pretend there is soap in your eyes. Or better, put it in for real. Smear soap in your eyes so it burns like a hot poker, and that will fool them and they won't even guess that you have heard them, and if you make them think they are not heard, then maybe they'll go away. But they won't go. They never go, don't you see?

You have to wrap your towel around the wet underwear and drip all the way to the phone, and you have to call your sister and say, "Hey, why don't you come on over, there's no one here, there's no one looking at me and I am fine. So it's a great day and why don't you come over?"

And you have to laugh and try not to cry when she sounds scared and asks if you are safe, and you can't say you aren't, so you keep saying, "It's a lovely day, how about a visit, eh? How about we get our kids to play together, eh? Eh?"

And you keep your hand over your eyes while you are talking and dripping because they have not left yet, and you can't let them see your soul, and you can't let them know that you know they are here to kill you.

Your sister says she'll be right there and then you have won. But no one really wins until you are in the psych ward, the place for rest, the place for sleep. No one wins until the drugs are heavy and your inner light is dimmed and you are thick and dark and safe from the faces and the voices and the reflective glass.

In the psych ward they feed you and you don't have to get dressed. If you are lonely or scared or tired of fighting the demons, you can make a plan and circle the halls, walking and muttering and telling the faces to leave you alone and be sure to say hello to Brenda because she's certified, too. Wave as you walk by, but don't break the rhythm, the pace of your walk, and don't forget to sing and laugh a little. And when the nurses ignore you, keep going, keep walking, and let the rhythm take you, and walk faster and faster until you are running and there is Brenda again and she doesn't like that you keep waving to her and she is screaming at you and you are flapping and smashing your own face and dreaming of smashing Brenda's. And there is a security guard and there is the male nurse who is strong enough to hold you on the floor and now you are in your room and they are feeding you the blue pills just one or three and that's not working so how about a shot in the behind, the warm one that stings and burns and then you sleep and you aren't lonely any more and the voices are gone and all that is left is the blackness, and you might think you are dead, but there is no light at the end of the tunnel, and that is how you know you are in a psych ward and not dead.

Give me the needle full of sleep. Dark and warm, sleep at last. *Ouch*. And oh, do you have something for this hole? This one. The one over my navel and under my ribs. Right here. The place where the demons slide their way into my chest . . . You don't see it? You. Don't. See-e-e-e . . .?

Don't you see? Don't you see how much work it is to get in here?

This is better than home, my sweet, because the baby isn't here to see me, and the guards won't let my hands do what the voices say I should do. And the guards won't let my hands do what I want to so badly—to end this hell because I know my body is broken. Mom is free and I want to be free, too—maybe find Mom and be with her. I can't find myself. I can't find me. Dana? My sweet? Don't cry, please don't cry. He's gone? Oh, Dad . . . it's you . . .

Hi, Dad, well, I'm in the hospital, yeah, and my husband is a pervert, and he's having an affair with the chiropractor. I know because when we went there, they went in a room and closed a door and that's okay because I'm in love with the intern—he's my soulmate, Dad. And Dad,

Dana wants me dead and I want to be dead, too, and I'm scared, Dad, and I can't find me. Oh Dad, please help me. I can't find me but don't cry, Dad. I'm in the hospital and it's the next best thing to suicide anyhow. And we are trying new drugs, Dad, and a new doctor and he's the best and this will work for me and then I'll go home and have a family and a real life and maybe even a job and it will all be okay. No, Dad. Don't cry, Dad. Okay, love ya, too, Dad. Yeah. Love ya.

I wake up stiff and swollen one day and I can't bend my fingers. Water, I hear them say. She's retaining water. I hurt all over from the water. My insides are tight and swollen. She's toxic. *I'm toxic?* They talk to each other because they're not allowed to talk straight to people like me with the multicoloured wrist bands.

Except for the intern. He studies me, my face, my body, and he talks nice. He invites me two or three times a day to the lounge. I sit on the couch. He kicks back in the chair and puts his feet on the coffee table and asks me about my life, my marriage, my libido. He reminds me of the boys in high school. He makes me think about who I used to be before I married a cheating, miserable pervert like Dana. The intern makes me red in the cheeks. "You're blushing." He laughs and puts his hands behind his head.

"I could make you blush, too," I say.

He teases. I tease back, and we go back and forth until the nurse knocks on the door. He won't see me again until the next nurse's shift.

Week one. No more lithium for her. Nope. Gotta clean her out, flush her with an IV. Try something else.

At six in the morning I borrow a phone book from the nurse's desk and call all of my friends and Dana's, too. I tell Jill that I am leaving Dana for the intern. The intern is smooth and when he walks down the hall his hair blows a little and I can smell his cologne and sometimes the emblem on his shirt winks at me and I know it is a sign and he is my soulmate.

Week two. She'll lose a kidney doing this.

The drugs are heavy and I am still high. I know now that Dana is evil. I should have listened to my mother. I should have listened when she told me that he was no good. I'm married, though, and I can't trash the marriage. It's not the kind of thing I would ever do. But I see the intern, and he knows now that I like him. He likes me, too. He's young and too stupid to understand bipolar. He actually thinks he can believe what I tell him. Can't he see the multicoloured bracelet?

Week three. The new one didn't take either? She'll wreck her liver. Give her a good flush, and we'll find another combo to work with. Yup, yup, I'll get right on that.

The intern and I have been together now for three weeks. It's not physical, but we both know what is going on here. We both know that this was meant to be. I draw self-portraits for him with my pencil crayons. They show lightning bolts coming from my palms and from my forehead. He understands me. He really understands me. He still likes to make me blush. He still likes to see me in the lounge. I'd kiss him, but that's not the sort of thing I do now.

Week four. Does she look to you like she's tipping over? At least she's calmed down. Well, let's let her go home if she doesn't flap this week. Gotta have the bed.

I can do this. I can be too sluggish to flap. I can forget about the intern. I play bingo. So many numbers and letters, though, so much to keep track of. I watch the O.J. Simpson trial and sigh in relief with everybody else on the ward when he is found not guilty. We have all thought of doing what he has done. It could have been me. Really, it could have been anyone, right? I go to the woodworking shop and make a toy train for James. His third birthday. He's going to love it. He'll be so proud of his mother. A real psych ward success story. Going home on four drugs and a wooden train. Look, James, Mommy's back! She falls asleep in the chair and drools and can't read and slurs her speech and Daddy and the babysitter do everything. But Mommy built you a train. Aren't you a lucky boy? Isn't it great to have Mommy home? James?

31

The tree outside the front window is dripping. A thousand million drips from a million billion leaves. And I can hear them all. Each one pouring down the branch onto the green and waxy fingerlings. Screeching along the fold onto the veiny tips where the pool begins and the droplet forms. Then crashing to the patio. Stronger than the wind, louder than the music and the voices, the dripping tree pounds the pavement with her tears.

Home is the condo unit I'm managing in trade for rent, and I've been home from the psych ward for a week. Or maybe a month. Or is it a lifetime? I don't know which. I don't want to know. I don't know anything any more, except that my life is tiresome, and my drugs aren't working as they should. I know I don't want to be here. I want out. I'm not worth saving, and even the tree knows it today. She weeps for me, for all the life I will not be living after today, when I will finally be with Mom.

I pour myself onto the fuzzy green armrest and drop onto the couch, gripping my head, gluing it together with the palms of my stiff hands. Each drip, each breath, every movement on the earth is a torture to me, and today I'm ready to find my way out of it. I'm ready.

The house is impeccable. Not a thing is out of place. I have attained a perfection in housekeeping that my mother could never match, perfection that makes the neighbour lady gasp and other women's husbands jealous. See that, Mom? Not just a stupid shag carpet, but everything. Perfect, Mom. Perfect!

"How is it that Autumn can keep house the way she does and take care of her son and still be the resident manager of a sixty-condo housing project?" they wonder as they shuffle down the walkway and out the front gate. Dana doesn't let on about any of my secrets. When the men come to visit, he is proud and calm.

"Yep, she's a pretty good housekeeper," he says. He doesn't tell them about last night or the other day. He just lets them think that I'm okay, he's okay. He is just like my father that way. This is what Dad did for Mom. But I won't put Dana through that. Not any more. Keeping the secrets. Not any more.

It's time for the truth, and when it is all out there, when I am cold and stiff and dressed to go, he will be relieved of this burden and everyone will say, What a good man Dana is. See how he lived with her. She was crazy and sick, and he protected her and kept the secret out of respect for her. Isn't it a relief now that he is free to find real happiness? He deserves better than she could ever have given him.

The men will pat him on the shoulder and offer their condolences and whisper to him that they know of a cute single girl who would love to be a mom to James. And the ladies will cry and say how sad it is and then go home to the sink full of dishes and the dirty carpet and realize that they are normal and Autumn wasn't, and it is okay if they can never get the house in order. Better a mess on the outside than inside. Fine. Perfectly fine with me if they use me as their excuse for keeping a dirty house.

Today I will make my own way out of my mess at last. I haven't yet decided how. But I will. I'm working at it.

My doctor has already restricted the number of pills that he will let me have at one time. So I know I can't take Grandpa's way. I'm not allowed to drive the car, so an accident is out of the question. And the school zone in the neighbourhood goes around the loop by the school and reaches farther than I can walk. All the drivers have to go slow, so I won't be able to throw myself in front of a fast-moving vehicle.

The kitchen knife is always an option, but what if Sunni brings James back before Dana gets here? They'll wander into the kitchen and find me in a pool of blood and that will surely be something that Jimbo will remember. I don't want Jimbo to remember me that way. Or any way.

I don't want my son to remember me at all.

That tree. I sink deeper, pressing my slouching rounded back into the fresh clean couch and stare out at the tree. She keeps the rain off the window, so the only proof of a downpour is her dance, swaying and rocking under the weight of the water and the wind. It is a beautiful thing, this crying tree. It's crying for me. The tree cries for me.

I hear music. In my head:

Where can I turn for peace? Where is my solace?
When other sources cease to make me whole . . .

An old hymn, one of my mother's favourites. It sweeps into my mind, not through my ears, but through the hole in my chest. This hole, gateway to my soul, is the entrance for demons and music and fear. It opens once a day now, sometimes twice. No drug, no sleep, can make me thick enough. And I am tired of it. The vulnerability, the torment, the constant intrusion.

I reach beside the couch and pull up my Bible. The Bible is thick and solid and heavy. I grab it and flop it open onto my chest and lie back. I clutch it to my chest, over the hole. I let my head drop onto the armrest. I know what this position of mine looks like. I've seen it so many times. I look a lot like Mom now. I thought I understood her before. I was wrong. I did not understand her. Today I understand her. Perfectly.

I am angry. Angry at God, angry at life. I want to end this so desperately. Send lightning, send fire. Just end this for me. End it.

I rip the Bible off my chest and heave it to the side. I rant and cry and flap and scratch myself. I rip at my hair and shake and rock and scream until I have no energy left. I don't want to be like my mom. But this is what we do, Grandpa and Mom and I. A tradition. Today is my turn.

One last look.

In the bathroom mirror my face is swollen from the beating I have given it. And there it is! I see it. The look of the terrified kitten. The monster me, the lonely and the lost. I'm not like Mom. I *am* Mom. I know now. I know . . .

It's time.

How did that go? She gathered her poetry, her journals, and pillow. She checked the hose, the map, the gas tank. She was so methodical, so purposeful.

The time has come.

Methodically, purposefully, I pick and pull at myself, getting the loose hairs off. I'll be clean when he finds me. Maybe behind the shower curtain. Lying in the tub. With the water on.

A quick run-through. To make sure the house is in order. Dana will come home to a clean house tonight. Bathroom? Spic and span. Bedrooms? Perfect.

The living room? No. There—the Bible is lying in the corner. I fumble to pick it up. A passage leaps off the page at me. The words stand off the paper bold and clear, all the others falling behind in a blur of ink and parchment.

I blink at it.

Read it. My Girl.

I'm having trouble concentrating today. I can't—

Read it.

Isaiah, Chapter 61:

The Spirit of the Lord God is upon me; because the Lord hath anointed me to preach good tidings unto the meek; he hath sent me to bind up the broken-hearted, to proclaim liberty to the captives, and the opening of the prison to them that are bound.

He's speaking to me. Broken heart, broken mind, broken body. Trapped, bound, captive in a prison I cannot escape.

To proclaim the acceptable year of the Lord, and the day of vengeance of our God; to comfort all that mourn.

Will you come again? Will you save me? Will you love me and my mom? Will you take me on your cloud and let me wash your feet with my tears?

To appoint unto them that mourn in Zion, to give unto them beauty for ashes, the oil of joy for mourning, the garment of praise for the spirit of heaviness; that they might be called trees of righteousness, the planting of the Lord, that he might be glorified.

Lord, I want that gift, trade my ashes for beauty, give me beauty for all my ashes and I will, Lord, I will stand tall, I'll be a tree for you with deep roots and strong branches. Is it too much to ask? Beauty for ashes?

I haven't read for months, because I couldn't. I could never understand the words, but I understand this passage at a glance. Again and again I read it. I feel its promise of relief and redemption. I sit back down on the couch and close my eyes. The voices and music are still with me, but I can reach beyond the front of my brain where they live. I go looking for her. I need her.

"Is it true?" I ask My Girl aloud. "Just tell me that it is so, and I will live to see this promise made real. Just say it is true."

Nothing.

No, there is something. I feel a sudden sense of peace.

I feel a sensation of floating.

I know I am still seated on the couch because I can look down and see the top of my head. But . . .

Not my own cropped, stubby dark hair. No, now my hair is long, hanging down my back, brushing across the tops of my shoulder blades. I am thin and beautiful, the way I used to be. I stand up, and I am standing tall, the way I used to, before I started hunching over.

"Can I?"

Yes.

"I want to try her body on me. Just for a minute."

Just for a minute, then.

Oh. Her body feels so good to me. This body is different from the one in the mirror. Different from the one in the shower stall. Strong, tight, confident, intelligent, sane, joyful, and abundantly blessed. I can feel all of these things. I feel the cool of a stone floor under my bare feet and notice the sensation of wearing blue jeans that fit without digging into my belly. Oh, and no voices! No voices in my head. And . . . *oh!*

I look down beside me and see a pretty little girl with blonde straight hair and wide eyes standing by my feet. She is looking into my face lovingly. She is not even a surprise to me.

"I know you," I say to her, and I can see she knows me as only a daughter can. "You're mine. My own little girl."

I want to scoop her up and hold her to me.

Not yet, says My Girl in the Back Brain. *Not yet.*

"Not yet? Does that mean . . .? There will be a yet? A girl after all? And a new me?"

Nobody answers my questions, not God, and not My Girl.

And yet . . .

I saw a new woman there. Me. Not the monster me, but . . . Dare I even say it? A normal me. I felt her feeling normal.

And the girl. My daughter. She looks like me. Oh, please, please, can she be mine?

More a reality than any delusion I've ever had. More a reality than one of my hallucinations. More than a vision. More than a joy.

This was a promise. From God.

And God wouldn't lie, doesn't lie, never lies. Somehow I have to live. To see the promise. To live the promise. It's not time after all. *The time has not come. God has promised.*

I run and look into a mirror. At the monster me, yes, with the swollen, blotched, freshly beaten face and the close-cropped hair, yes, that monster, but the monster with a new look in her eyes. Is that a look of hope? Of life? Of joy? Can I even dare to hope for a life of joy?

32

Dad found a new job in Cardston, working as the maintenance manager for a group of church buildings. He was still poverty-stricken, with Barb and Jennifer now added to his list of mouths to feed. There was no engineering work in Cardston, but he couldn't bring himself to leave Mom's dream house. So he continued to live in her nightmare.

Trapped in that house, he obsessed about the madness that had taken Mom; he thought about it incessantly, praying, studying, fasting, reading, searching. But now, besides me and Mom, he had another trial to endure.

My brother Joey started showing some of the signs—the attention deficit, the restlessness, the confusion. He had been so soft and innocent and easygoing before the illness took him. But now Joe was thirteen, stocking weapons, painting his face black, and whipping chains around in the streets, pounding spikes through his bedroom door. He cycled from rages to depression to mania. He was diagnosed, he was medicated. His life was over, and Dad knew it. Joe was stuck in the familiar family pattern. The whole household was afraid of Joe. I cried when I heard that.

Dad must have cried, too. But he decided that tears were not enough. He had to act. Denial could not hide this. Not again. Not with his children. Not with his son. Under the same roof where Mom had lived until she took her life. He could not stand by and watch Joe take this all-too-familiar trek to suicide. He had to do something. Moved by faith and outrage and love and fear, he vowed to save his children from the madness. He all but gave up his own life, dedicating himself to saving mine and Joe's. He had faith that we could be cured. He was incensed that drugs and the medical profession could do so little.

He redoubled his effort to understand our illness. More than that, he began an impossible quest for its cure. For months he searched and talked and studied and read. From a distance, he must have looked mad himself, poring over medical books, taking up residence in the local university library, and combing the Internet. A boiler engineer taking on a mental illness that continued to baffle all of medicine? Poor Tony, what on earth does he think he can do? He won't talk about anything else, eh? Absurd.

Even I felt bad for him. What could he do? He might as well have been looking for the fountain of youth in the frozen Yukon. Preposterous.

Preposterous to all but Anthony Stephan, my loving dad, trying to find the right answer, just as he did at the kitchen table on the acreage. My dad, whose mission in life was now to save ours.

"Autumn. Are you okay?"

I am weak, and the phone is heavy and cold against my drug-flushed face. "No, Dad. I'm not."

"What's going on? I've been thinking about you. Are you doing any better?"

"No. Got really high, had to take some drugs to come down."

"Are you safe? Is Dana taking care of you?"

"He's fine." There is a long silence. Dad breathes into the phone, and I am dull and I don't care if he's worried.

"I made a new friend. David Hardy. He's up there visiting his kids, and I gave him your address. He's coming over to your place tonight with some calcium and some vitamins."

"What? What?"

"I just want you to take them."

"No. I can't have company today. I'm sick today."

"Sweetie, he's coming over. You let him talk to you. You take the vitamins. I mean it. You do it. Just do it. Please. For me."

"Whatever, Dad. Dana can decide." I am rude on my sedatives. I am mean and uncaring and I talk as if I'm drunk. I hate myself on these drugs. But I need the drugs to stay off the ceiling and out of the bars. I need the drugs to keep me living with Dana and James. If it weren't for the drugs, I'd really be gone. I know it.

David comes over, just as Dad said he would. He brings his son-in-law with him. They are two soft-spoken men, barely loud enough to hear across the kitchen table. The Ativan has worn off and I am back to being agitated. I cannot sit still, and I cannot listen to them for long. Dana sits and they talk about the supplements David has brought over. I kneel on my kitchen chair. I tap on the table. My Girl tells me to stop acting like a jerk, but I just can't find a way to be polite. I bounce my bum on my heels, and then I give up and stand up and pace around the kitchen until they leave.

Dana has three new pills for me to take several times a day. I swallow them. And I am no better for it. The days pass slowly, painfully. I am waiting for my miracle. Waiting for the fulfillment of a promise. It's hopeless. Hope will never come.

It is midnight. I take a belt sander to our dining room table. Before long, sawdust and grit and brass filings decorate the pale pink carpet. I paint the table teal and blue with streaks of white. I call it marbling.

But all the sandpaper and paint and frenzied mess won't satisfy my racing mind, so I sit at my handiwork and shake and cry and flap until Dana finds me and tries to get me to come back to bed. I won't go. He offers me several Ativan. Four more than usual.

Ativan. He's trying to kill me again. I run for my life. I hide in the bedroom. I lock him out and call Dad, who lives six hours to the south. I beg him to come and save me from the killer, my husband.

"He's not a killer, Autumn."

"He is a killer. I can't, I can't. Oh help me, Dad, save me, save me. I can't."

"What, Autumn, what can't you do?"

"I can't find me, Dad. I'm lost, Dad. I'm dying, Dad. I can't find me."

I hear the door rattling. Dana is using a nail to unlock it. I scream. The neighbours can hear. They are used to this by now.

"Ahhhhhh! I'm dying, he's a killer, I can't find me."

"Hey, kiddo, don't worry, I found the answer."

"What?"

"Yeah, I found the missing ingredients. We've got the answer!" Now I remember. I've already tried his cockamamie ideas about nutrition. Three months should have done it.

"It works. We added a liquid, a bunch of trace minerals. Joe stopped taking his drugs today."

"You can't do that. Are you nuts?"

"You go to a hospital and be safe."

"You're crazy."

"You just let Dana take you to the hospital, and I'll come get you later. We'll do the same thing for you as we did for Joe and you'll be okay, honey."

"You can't take Joe off his meds. He'll die. Are you stupid? He'll die!"

"You'll be okay."

Now Dana is in the room, and I have to fight him. I drop the phone and punch and kick and he takes it. I spit and scream until I am tired, then I cry and moan. He holds me tight and tells me that I'll feel better soon and hauls me to the car. He belts me in and uses the child lock on the door so I can't get out, and he drives. I see him from the side, the tears rolling down his face. He is weeping openly and I am sorry he's crying, but he's still a killer and doesn't deserve my pity. My Girl cries, too. But I don't. I am dark and empty. The hole in my chest is wide open and I feel nothing. Nothing. I sit in the seat, strapped tight, and I don't fight to get out. We pass bright neon signs and roll under the streetlights, warm and yellow, flashing and fading across the car, lighting across Dana's face, glinting off his tears, his wet nostrils.

I am back in a hospital, and I am blank.

This time I stay under watch in the suicide room, the one with the short toothbrushes, just plastic stubs with soft bristles—too short to sharpen, too small to choke on. The room with the outlets covered in flat plastic screwed on tight.

I don't play bingo this time or do crafts. I don't call my friends at six in the morning to tell them stories about my evil husband or the gorgeous intern. In fact, the intern isn't gorgeous. He's moved to a new ward, but when he comes to touch my shoulder in the hall and to say hello, I hardly recognize him. I wonder what I ever saw in him. I am flat and dark, and he is visibly turned off by my new voice, my new face. There is no spark in me for him and I do not blush with his touch. I don't blush for anyone any more.

I don't watch TV. I just lie in bed and think about getting out of here so I can ditch this broken body and be with Mom. We understand each other at last. The intern taught me the last thing I needed to know about forgiving Mom. High tides always bring soulmates. Yeah, Mom and I will get along just fine now. *Hear that, Mom? Just you and me now.*

Maybe I have it all wrong. The promise won't come true in this life but in the next. Yeah, that's it. New body, new baby, all my dreams fulfilled in the new life. The promise was not a reason to go on living. Rather, it was a reason for dying.

When I checked out a week later, I was on a five-drug cocktail. Haldol, Rivotril, Ativan, Epival, and Cogentin. I sat in the doctor's office in and out of sleep, drooling down my chin. It didn't matter. The doctor was talking to Dana anyway. They never talked to me now.

I was never to be left alone with James. Dana had to give me round-the-clock adult supervision. He promised to get help from his parents and from my dad. Those were the conditions of my release. Dana promised.

I heard the doctor tell him, Just give me a couple of years, and we'll find a balance for Autumn. Be patient. There's a combination some-where that will work for her.

I remember thinking a single crystal-clear thought, one brief sparkle through the stupor. A couple of years?

Didn't they say that two years ago?

33

"**H**i, Mom Stringam," I called out as I stumbled through the front door. I kicked off my shoes and propped open the door for Dana, loaded up with clothing bags and toys. He walked in and stopped to breathe deeply, sucking in the warm yeasty smell of fresh bread.

"Oh, Mama, that smells awesome." Dana missed his mom's fresh bread and wholesome meals. As a girl raised in the southern part of Utah in a tiny farming community, she had learned the arts of baking and sewing and making do with whatever her father gleaned from the land. In the harsh Canadian north she applied everything she knew to the establishment of a beautiful, successful, busy home.

James burst through the front door. He ran straight downstairs to find his favourite toy. As he skidded around the corner of the wide carpeted staircase, Mom Stringam came around from the upstairs kitchen. She stood at the top of the stairs wiping her hands on a clean towel. She was so neat and prim in her blue-checked cotton apron and a carefully curled short haircut. The cordless phone was pressed between her shoulder and ear.

"Just a minute," she said into the phone. "Come on in, guys. Dana, you can take that stuff straight downstairs if you want to." She seemed enthusiastic enough. She looked right at me and smiled her sweet tipped-to-the-side smile. No condemnation in her, although she knew my story all too well. Her strong jawline came to a point as she smiled, reminding me of Dana and every other one of her seven kids.

Dana took our things downstairs, and Mom Stringam turned back into the kitchen. I decided to go for drama. I crawled up the twelve stairs to the front hall. I probably could have walked, but my legs did burn with fatigue. Besides, I needed to show her that I was not well enough to help with the meal. She never expected much of me anyway. But I had to be sure that she got it. *Autumn's a bit odd, you know.* It never occurred to me that she'd had this idea for a while. *What's to get? You've been odd ever since she met you.*

I got to the top and rose up on my knees, facing the front room. The Stringam house was elegant. It was full of wooden treasures and vases and dolls from other countries to which they had travelled. There was a fine hand-woven floral rug in the living room, and all of the décor picked up the colours of the rug, jewelled teal and gentle pink and cream. The furniture was light and soft, except for the hand-carved and brass-laden cherrywood rocking chair in the corner and the matching cherrywood coffee table on the centre of the woven rug. Behind the rocking chair and all around the room were lush ferns, blossoming trees, and short exotic, leafy plants. Even on a cold and dark day, this room was bright and airy. It would do just fine.

"Oh, your legs are bothering you again," Mom Stringam said in her sincere and sympathetic tone as she came from the kitchen to greet me. "Well, don't worry about helping with supper. You just go relax in the living room, and I'll have it on the table in no time."

"Grandma!" James had found his truck and made his way up the plush carpeted stairs as quickly as his diapered torso could travel. "I got da truck!" Everything James said to his grandma was done with a loud voice and a big smile. She paid special attention to him. I could see he felt safe when she was around. *Good.* He would do just fine here, later, when it was time.

"Come here, my big boy," Mom Stringam said as she stooped to his eye level and wrapped him in her arms for a long tickly hug. It was good that they loved each other. They'd be spending lots of time together soon.

Dinner was great. Crisp green salad, warm casserole, fresh-baked white bread, and an apple pie, big and brown and as rumpled as the foothills.

"So how was your day, Dad?" Dana asked.

"Oh, I don't know . . . pretty busy. I—"

"Mine, too," I said, cutting Dad Stringam off mid-sentence. "I woke up with a plan to redo the dining room. I flipped all the chairs and tore off the old upholstery. I've got four chairs to work on, so I have to get more of the matching material to make the skirts for them, and then I decided to cover the cushion on the rocker—you know, the rocker by the fireplace—"

"Autumn took out the belt sander the other night and stripped the top of our dining room table," said Dana. "She's really into interior decorating."

—He forgot to say, *And then she beat on me, and I wrestled her into a vehicle, and she spent a week in the psych ward . . .* Always another side to the story, eh? A voice slithers into the front of my brain.

I plead with the voice for privacy: *Shhh, that part's a secret.*

"Yeah, I found a magazine and went on the Internet to get marbling designs, and I'm painting a marble effect on the table so it will look like one giant slab. Then I just have to figure out the way to fill in the groove in the side of it from where I tore out the brass ribbing. You wouldn't have brass ribbing in a marble slab, so it's gone. I think I'm going to fill in the groove with putty and then just paint over it. Did you know about the yarn sale at Lewiscraft, Mom? It's awesome, but the stuff on sale isn't as nice as the really soft, fluffy sweater yarn, so I got a bunch of that to work on a crochet pattern I am designing. Oh yeah, that reminds me of the doily on your toilet top—it's crocheted like the kind that my mom's friend used to make, but she did a whole tablecloth that looked like a picture of *The Last Supper* when it was done. She could crochet without even looking! I can, too, but my hands are stiff from the Haldol, y'know, so my fingers ache pretty bad after a few minutes of crocheting, and that's why I am starting to paint more instead. I am going to paint a big mural on James' bedroom wall as soon as I get done refinishing his bed and dressers, but I can't do that until I stop the Haldol because it makes my knees hurt."

I shovel large bites of food into my mouth. I chew and talk and spit chunks of apple pie. I am fully aware that I am dominating the conversation at the table; I am even embarrassed by it. I wish that I could just slow down. It isn't fun being the only one talking, but I still can't get my motormouth to take a break.

I have to talk. The voices are coming back, and I need to talk fast enough and loud enough so that I can drown them out.

—*Mom Stringam wants you dead*, the voices tell me.

Oh, no! Her, too? "And then my bedroom is next, that old dresser needs some lovin'. . ."

—*Did you see her roll her eyes when Dana said you used the belt sander?*

No, she didn't roll her eyes. My Girl is here. Good girl, help me out.

—*She did, and she wants Dana to marry a new girl and she hates you and she wishes that Dana had never met you.*

She does? "We have the vanity and the highboy and the headboard, they all need to be stripped . . ."

No, she does not.

—*You aren't good enough for him. You are low class and your family is wrecked and you don't fit in here.*

I should go. ". . . the mirror, I'd like to have it replaced . . ."

They are lying. Just you stay put.

—*Look at her. She's not looking when you talk. That's because she wants you dead.*

It's true, she isn't looking at me, it's true. How will I spend the night under the care of a woman who wants to kill me?

—*Check your food.*

Is she poisoning me? "This pie is great!"

The food is just fine. Stop poking the pie, it's fine.

Dana reaches under the table and grips my thigh. Both of my legs have started a wild involuntary shake, and he knows that my agitation is mounting. He knows the voices are back. The table is shaking and the glasses are clinking against the edges of the plates.

"She's gonna blow!" Dana laughs. His smile breaks the tension. Everyone chuckles. Even I manage a quick snorting laugh before I get back to my babble. Dana is squeezing my thigh hard. He's afraid to leave me. He's afraid for them.

"So I have to get going for midnight shift, guys," he says. "Thanks for taking care of my little family for me. Hopefully, things will settle down for Autumn in a day or so, so that she can sleep at home again."

"Don't worry about it, honey." Mom Stringam leans over and puts her hand on Dana's shoulder.

"Thanks, Mama."

He turns to me. "Okay, love doll, I have to go." The words come in one long sigh of resignation. "Here, you take my ring so I don't lose it at work." Dana hands me his wedding band. It is smooth, rounded, and wide. A very plain gold reminder of the covenant we made before he knew what he was getting into.

—He's leaving his ring because he's going to a bar. He's not going to work. He's going out all night to look for a woman who's better than you. The voices are yelling now.

Is that true?

No! He doesn't drink and he just called you love doll. They are liars. Stop listening.

Okay.

Dana touches my shoulder to bring me back from my blurry-vision staring at the wall. "Your meds. You've got some water in your cup." His ring is still in my hand. I slip my wedding rings off and put his ring on first. My engagement ring is just big enough to keep Dana's ring from slipping past and off my finger. His large ring dangles between the base of my finger and my engagement ring, and I give my hand a shake to see that it is secure. I shake it again a few times. *And a few times more.* Until Dana snatches my hand and holds it to break the pattern.

He kisses the top of my head. "Love Only, babe. I'll see you tomorrow afternoon." I nod and smile and swallow my fistful of pills.

Mom Stringam cleans up the dishes and helps James get into bed upstairs. By the time she is finished, I am melting into the couch in the living room. The drugs are doing what they do best. I feel absolutely nothing. Still, in the nothingness, a quick vibration in the front of my head is looming. *Weird.* That's not how it works. I form a thought, and it surprises me. Usually by now the meds have stopped my thoughts, stopped the racing thoughts, stopped thought altogether. *No thoughts.*

"Freaky."

"What is freaky, dear?"

Mom Stringam is standing in front of me.

"Oh. Nothing. I'm usually asleep by now."

"Oh."

"But my head just keeps on going."

"Well, rest would be a good thing, so why don't you go get ready, and I'll tuck you in, in a few minutes."

"Yeah. Sleep would be a good thing."

But sleep will not come. I toss and fluff my pillow too many times. I scratch my nose and get stuck in the pattern of scratching until it hurts, and My Girl screams in my head, *Stop it, just stop it!*

—*Yeah, stop scratching*, chimes a slippery voice from the front of my head. *Believe me, honey, your face is the only thing you have going for you right now. Don't wreck that.*

Mom Stringam pokes her head in the room to check on me, but I am well under the covers. She doesn't see the tears on my face or the sweat on my pillow. She slips out and closes the door.

I awaken. The house is dark and quiet. I am so alert, so agitated, so . . . up!

Oh no, the meds aren't working. I'm going up on the tide. A swinging little song comes to me. It isn't one that I've heard before. It's just a make-it-up-as-you-go song.

Up, up, up, up, going to the top, up, up . . . So jazzy. I just can't hold still. *Yeah yeah yeah yeah, blah blah blah blah blah bu-blah.* My head is rocking on the pillow and I am thrashing under the blankets. I thrash for minutes. Or maybe hours. Thrashing and thrashing.

I awaken the next morning exhausted. My pillow is soaked, my hair wet. And I am shaken by a residual image in my front brain. Burned there, set deep in my tissue. I know now. I know why murderers kill and rapists rape. I know how people hurt their babies and ravage themselves. I understand the darkest evils of human behaviour. What part was a dream? What parts actually happened? The jumping. Dancing. Thrashing, thrashing. Maybe none of it. Maybe all. Maybe more than I know.

I am so tired. I sleep the morning away, face down on the carpet in a sunny spot, bathed in the warmth of the front room. The morning medication fills in what is left of the hole in my chest, and I feel nothing but the heat of the sun on my back. My mind goes nowhere and remembers nothing except the weight of a secret dream, a sick reality, a knowledge that I am never going to be okay. Never. Knowing what I know, that I am evil. Whether I dreamt last night or whether I lived it, last night was too sick to live through again. I don't want to live it any more, either in my dreams or in my body.

"Autumn, are you crying?" Mom Stringam has heard my heavy breathing and whining. I lift my head, leaving my snot and tears in her carpet.

"I'm just so stinking sick of it, Mom. I'm twenty-two and as good as dead." I can't tell her the scary stuff, the last-night stuff. She will be afraid of me. She sits on the floor by my head and puts her fingers in my hair. She caresses my scalp and face and blends her tears with mine. She cries with me. Or for me. Or for her son and grandson.

Her tears are fake, of course. She wants me dead.

Dana asks for his ring in the afternoon.

I don't know what to tell him.

"I had a pretty bad nightmare."

"And?"

"And the ring was just gone when I woke up."

We search my pockets, the bedroom, the house. We don't find the ring. I'm sick about it.

I slip into the bathroom to steal a moment with My Girl.

"Where is it? Did you watch me last night?"

She doesn't answer.

"C'mon, I need the ring. Did you see where it ended up?"

She answers, though not in so many words. Instead she floods me with a vision, *that vision*. Of the night before, the dance, the whipping and splashing, the vomit, the shower. She lets me hear the sound of the gold bouncing off the walls, the windows, the toilet. The sounds and sights and no more. She won't talk to me. She looks away. At the very time I need her most, even My Girl betrays me.

I mourn the loss of Dana's ring. I mourn the loss of my mind. Most of all I mourn the loss of My Girl.

So. This is it. The place they call rock bottom. She has led me here and left me here with nothing left to lose.

I can not, will not, live without her. I will take care of this once and for all. Later. After I have a nap. After I get over being so desperately tired.

34

Where am I?

I wake to the smell of roast beef and steaming vegetables, so I know it's a safe place, but where? The room is dark, lit only by warm light splayed under the door. My feet are hot, twisted in my nylons that have migrated around my legs. I remember moments of being hot, twisting in a restless sleep. But where the heck am I? I struggle to get off the bed, bleary and heavy and confused. It's all I can do to sit up. I take a moment to rest, to listen for a clue. I hear voices, adults laughing. They seem familiar, family, but I can't decide who. I hear children. They are running overhead and thumping down carpeted stairs. That rattle! I have it at last. The spiral staircase that rattles and creaks and bumps when the kids hop down each step. I recognize the noise. I am in Dad's house. I remember. Today is Sunday. I remember Dana left last night. I remember I am tired of being babysat. I want to go home, to my own home. I have lost so much on these drugs. Weekdays. Weekends. Entire vacations.

I remember now. This morning. Not a good start to the day. I had to walk out of church early. I could not be still. I tried to sit still, tried to endure the meeting, but no. The energy kept welling up inside me, and the voices were too angry, and I was almost flapping when Dad noticed and led me out. He took me by the shoulders, a firm grip, a grip not to say no to. I let myself be held in his strong hands as we walked out, I fighting back the urge to flap, Dad smiling—It's all right, it's all right—to answer the weak, knowing smiles of the members of the congregation.

Back at his house Dad gave me some Ativan and led me to this room.

I dumped myself into bed. I remember now. He gave me a fistful of his pills and a sip of some nasty liquid. There's a story to these pills. I can't remember the story. Just that they make me angry and I call them pig pills, but I didn't fight about it. I just went to sleep.

And now I am here and I am hungry and there are voices outside this room that I don't recognize. I cannot be friendly today. I cannot be civil. So I won't go to see.

I sit on the edge of the bed, in the dark, until my stomach can't ignore the smells. I'm hungry more than fearful, more than shy, more than anything else. I stand up, wait a moment for my head to clear, and shuffle from the bed to the door. I let in the rest of the light and slip from the bedroom like a shadow. I wish nobody would notice me. I take the only empty seat at the table. Maybe they won't notice. Maybe they'll just let me be. Maybe—

"Autumn, you woke up." Dad seems so pleased to notice the obvious.

I give him a weak smile.

"This is Bill."

"Hi, Bill."

"Good to meet you, Autumn."

"Bill is a psychiatric nurse."

"Oh."

It's not as if I haven't met one before. Dad has chosen his company carefully today. I eat my dinner and the conversation carries on as though I am not here. But I do not go unnoticed. Bill is watching me. Lively storytelling, lots of laughter. Dad and Barb are enjoying themselves. Bill acts as if he's right in the mood with them, but he's ever watchful of me, ever noticing. I intend to stay quiet, giving him nothing to notice, but as soon as I announce the intention to myself, it is tested.

I feel it coming on, like hot tar welling up from my bowels into my throat, bubbling and churning. First the agitation, then thoughts of Mom. Her death. The abandonment, the anger, the grief, the voices, the hole. I can't take it. I can't take it. I can't.

I am flapping, screaming, out of my chair, into the kitchen. I lunge for the drawers, rummaging for a knife. There are none to be found. Dad knows better.

Dad is pulling me away from the drawer, the nice family dinner now a scene out of *Who's Afraid of Virginia Woolf?*

"Autumn." Dad holds me up in that familiar bear hug. He's not angry with me for ruining the dinner, of course. This house is used to these kinds of outbursts and antics. After all, Mom lived here, and they have all been through a year of psychotic Joseph.

He knew it would come to this. Why else do you invite a psych nurse? Above all, I knew it would come to this. It always does. I hate it. I hate it, but I can't stop it.

"Let me go. I don't want to live like this." I am already hoarse from screaming. "Just let me go, Dad, just let me go."

Dad holds me, and Bill holds my arms down, away from my face. I don't know him and I don't want him touching me. Soon they are force-feeding me Ativan and a handful of other pills. I am gagging on the taste of sulphur in the liquid, that new supplement they're giving me. I hate it. I sputter, claw, scream. The fight doesn't end until the Ativan begins to work. I give up.

Today I will not die. I'll just sleep, and that's the next best thing. Back in the room, my nylons are still on, but I can't care. I drop onto the bed and let the drugs take me back to that other world, the place where I live now, where hell has no boundaries and all of my darkest imaginings are the truth.

From the bed I can hear their voices again, in the kitchen. They are not laughing now. I can't hear what they're saying, but by the tone I know. They are worried. Now even Dad is afraid that the new supplement isn't going to work. Bill is saying I'd be better off back on a ward. Again.

I don't care now. The Ativan creeps through my mind, ridding me of my will to act out. I want to sleep, but sleep doesn't come. I lie paralyzed, haunted by visions of death and carnage, a hundred different scenes, and every victim is me. I am guilty, I am lost, and I am so alone, unable to move, unable to rise, to run, to save myself, to be saved. Finally the sleep comes between me and my desperation. Finally. Maybe tomorrow I'll kill myself.

Monday morning Dad wakes me up. I take the supplements from his hand before I am awake enough to argue about the size of the pills and the taste of the liquid. I take my drugs, too. And I sleep again.

"What is that stuff?" I ask the next time Dad comes in with the bottles of pills and the bitter liquid and a cup of water for washing everything down. It's like swallowing a fistful of marbles in spoiled vinegar.

"It's just vitamins and minerals, completely natural stuff. No drugs. Do you like it?"

"Yeah, it's okay." Except for the taste. And the number of pills. And the size of them.

I sleep again.

Each time I awake, it is because Dad wakes me. He comes home from work several times to feed me more of the supplement. He leaves, I sleep. Oh, how I sleep. All day long. The sleep is deep and thick as a down comforter. I am wrapped in it, barely able to move. My speech is slurred, my head boggy. My right eye will not stay open, no matter how much I lift my brow and pull at my lids with my fingers.

It is a struggle just to sit up. I fall asleep at the table, on the couch, on the toilet, in Dad's hug on the way to the bedroom. I finally decide to stay in bed, immobilized by the black downy sleep that will not retreat.

"Are you okay?" Dad comes in to sit on the edge of the bed. He has my night meds and my supplements. Night already. My, how time flies.

"Not all right. Can't stay awake. Hmmm. Know what?"

"What?"

"I didn't swing today."

"You didn't?"

"No. Every day, usually, I get my hole in my chest, and the voices come, but today I just slept and there was no hole." It felt like a long speech for my thick tongue to make.

"I think it's working." I hear hope in his voice, and excitement. "Why do you think you are so tired, Autumn? Why do you think that is?"

"I don't know. Maybe I just need the sleep."

I take the handful of pills from him and swallow hard. So many pills and so big. Was it necessary to take so many? I go to sleep feeling something new. Hope? *Not that again.*

Tuesday I awaken on my own. I don't get out of bed right away. Just lie there feeling it. Something is different. I wait, with my eyes closed. Am I dead? I wiggle my toes. Not dead. And my feet are not in the nylons any more. I smell the blankets: generic laundry detergent. So this is still Dad and Barb's house. Winter sunlight pours through the window, warm on my face, bright on my eyelids. And I am not myself. My eyes are closed, but there is no image of my death, no bloody gore, no dark sexual violence, no live dissection or murder of myself.

I push my arms under the blankets to feel my chest. There is no hole. Just me, in bed, with a mid-morning sun on my face, no portal for demons to slide into my chest.

I open my eyes and listen. I can hear someone moving in the kitchen. I stop in the bathroom on the way to the kitchen and look in the mirror. My face is still fat and my mascara is still smeared from yesterday, but there is a change, something about the way I see myself. Something. But what?

Right off, Dad sees a difference in me, too.

"Wow, Autumn, you are looking better." Dad. Always hopeful. I just saw myself in the mirror, Dad. You're overstating the case—two times over.

"Look, Barb, her eyes are open."

"Wow, that's great, eh?"

"Yeah." Both eyes open. Call a press conference.

Dad is so excited, but I don't want to get his hopes up. "I feel okay."

We sit down to breakfast and eat together. Barb has made fried-egg sandwiches on toast with bacon and onions on the side. I eat the food, grateful that someone is taking care of me.

It occurs to me that I have not been taking care of myself. "I think I'll have a shower this morning."

"Really?" Dad smiles.

I take my morning meds and Dad's pile of supplements. As they take hold of me, I don't want the shower after all. So sorry, Dad. I fall asleep for the rest of the day.

When Dad comes home to give me my mid-afternoon dose of supplements, he awakens me and watches me choke them down. I wait for the rest of it.

"What?" he says.

"My meds?"

"No drugs, Autumn. You don't need them any more."

"Dad." It isn't merely that I have heard that kind of thing before. I have said it so many times myself. Dad, that's what all the nice bipolar people say. "I can't do it, Dad. I'm not allowed to stop—"

"You have to. You're stoned."

"I can't, Dad. You know what Dana said when he left me here. I can't mess with my meds."

"You're going to have to stop taking them if you're ever going to be normal. Haven't you felt a change, Autumn?"

I give him a stare of disbelief. Dad, I'm a manic-depressive. Change is nothing to me. Change *is* me. Day-to-day, hour-to-hour, minute-to-minute change. Just like Mom. "You are feeling better already, aren't you?"

Well . . . "The visions have stopped."

"Then you don't need the drugs any more."

"My head is still racing."

"That will end. Give it time."

It's the first time anybody has ever suggested I could be well without the psychotropic drugs. I know I will never wake up if I keep taking them. And it's Dad, not me. He's the one giving me permission. So I try it.

On Wednesday I skip the morning dose of drugs altogether and shock everyone by staying up.

"How are you feeling?" Dad asks as he sits down for lunch.

"Good," I say. "My hole is closed up."

"What do you mean?"

"My hole—the hole in my chest. It's been closed since yesterday morning. I am solid now. I feel like I am totally solid."

Dad sits and stares at me for a bit, his eyes both hopeful and fearful. And damp. "Yeah, it's working."

I'm not so sure. I try to sound sure for him, but I am not sure enough of the miracle to risk taking a shower. Dana is even less sure than I am.

I sit on the countertop in the kitchen and tell him the news over the phone.

"What? Stop the drugs? No, I don't think so, hon. Dr. G. said not to rock the boat."

"But my hole is closed up." My lips quiver.

"No, hon, you are not going to do this."

"They just make me sleep all of the time, Dana. I don't need the drugs any more."

"Bull. Let me talk to your dad."

I hear only Dad's end of the conversation: "They have her so loaded up on that crap, she can't even open her eyes . . . I know I haven't been living with her, but I am now . . . I know it's been only three days . . . You have to see her . . . Has it been working? . . . Then what do you have to lose? . . . Hey, I already lost *my* wife . . ."

They were both desperate, each in his own way. Dad wanted to believe in the miracle so I could be saved from my mom's fate. Dana wanted to believe, too, but he was afraid that he'd lose me again to the madness if the miracle failed. In the end they came to a compromise. I stopped taking Haldol, Rivotril, Ativan, and Cogentin that day. I would keep taking the Epival until Dana was convinced I was stable.

On Thursday I took a shower. Alone. With the door closed. With all my clothes off. A shower. For Dad, a breakthrough. For me, a miracle at last.

35

Dana met us about halfway home. I was glad to switch cars and be with him. I did my best to control my mouth, to look sane, and for a change it wasn't that tough to do. I felt solid and optimistic, but I felt something else, too. A new kind of panic was growing inside me. Not the visions or the voices, not the high-speed thoughts and racing out-of-control creativity. Not the destructive mental depression. This panic was different. It was in my body, not my mind. I couldn't tell Dana about it. He'd think my miracle was a mirage. He'd say I was sick and put me back on the meds.

Saturday passed with only moderate mood swings. Sunday went by without any problems. But we avoided church, just to be safe. I had gone six days now without visions or voices or holes. But I was not sleeping.

"Dana." I am writhing even as I wake up. I am squirming and pushing my legs against the sheets like a kid digging in the sand with her heels. A perpetual motion fed by the grinding hunger inside me. "I can't breathe, I can't breathe."

"Lie still, hon."

"My heart. I think I'm having a heart attack."

"Stop kicking."

"I can't."

He reaches over to pull me toward him. "Oh crap, hon, you're soaked."

"It's sweat." I'm shaking inside. "I'm sick. Ohhhh, you gotta help me."

"Do you need an Ativan?"

"Yeah."

"Where are they?"

I have stashed an emergency supply in the bathroom cabinet. "Right next to the cough syrup."

He gets up. He hesitates.

"Hurry."

He looks at me strangely.

"What?"

"You aren't babbling. You're not manic."

"I know."

"Autumn, this isn't you."

Not the old flapping me, anyhow. My hands are tight against my chest. Dana lies on his side and runs his hand up and down my back.

"Dana. My heart. I think I'm having a heart attack. It's beating like—" I begin to hack.

"Are you going to puke?"

Hack-hack-hack.

"Get up, get up, get up. Don't puke here."

I barely make it to the toilet. He comes into the bathroom and wipes my mouth clean on a towel.

"Make this stop, Dana—please, you have to help me."

"I know what this is."

"Then make it stop."

"It's withdrawal. You're addicted to your meds. I've heard the guys at work talk about coming off crack like this. You aren't sick."

"I just puked. That's not sick?"

"That's withdrawal. I'm not going to give you any Ativan."

"Please, just one."

"No."

I cried and shook and gripped my chest until the early hours of the morning. Yes, I'd had nights like this before on the way to getting sick. But never on the road to getting healthy.

Soon the "discontinuation syndrome" set in. Diarrhea, gut pains, and insomnia. As I started to lose the weight I had gained on the drugs, I experienced flashes of the feelings I'd had on the meds.

I began reading articles in alternative health magazines about drug withdrawal and cleansing. I began to learn about natural health remedies.

I was afraid to go back to my new doctor, the psychiatrist. I feared he would not believe me, that he might take my claims of wellness as a challenge and slap another multicoloured bracelet on me. Instead, I talked to my first doctor, my family doctor. He hadn't seen me since my first hospitalization. He was impressed with my recovery. He said the natural supplements made some sense. After all, everything we eat does something to alter our chemistry. But he said the drugs could not be affecting me long-term. Book knowledge, not my body's knowledge. Apparently, he'd forgotten to read the part about discontinuation syndrome when he learned his drugs. That or maybe my body's knowledge wasn't common knowledge just yet. And I was okay with that. I didn't feel so dependent on him for answers any more.

I wasn't so dependent on anybody. I began to develop a mind of my own. A mind free of voices, floating faces, and fear. And gradually, I began to trust my recovery, to believe in my stability. Waking in the morning was no longer a gamble, a guessing game of who I would be. I began to understand myself, to find my core personality. I cooked and read and listened to music. I did the laundry, took showers, and went to restaurants with Dana.

And I started finding strange things in my home, like the collection of new knitting yarn, a thousand dollars' worth at least. Before it had seemed normal to have heaps of yarn, still in the plastic bags, fresh from the store, pressed into shelves from floor to ceiling—a full walk-in closet packed with yarn. And I don't even knit! Behind the yarn I found paint, oil pastels, sandpaper, thread and more thread, bags of thread and bags of toothpicks, stencils, beads galore, tiny pieces of foam, bits of cloth, and reams of cloth. Behind that a mountain of coloured paper, stamps, pencils, a calligraphy set complete with instructions that I had never opened, stickers, and glue. Dozens of types for every possible use. Glue, glue, glue. What was I going to do with this stuff? What had I ever planned to do with it?

I was embarrassed when I realized how strange my life had been: the collections, the empty bank account, the filthy secrets of hidden psychosis scrawled on papers and stuffed in drawers and closets and boxes. Once I had called them journals; now I could see they were nothing more than rant, miserable memories of voices and visions and uncontrollable mania. I gathered the kits and supplies and gave them to a couple of local women's groups. Garbage bags full of brand-new yarn went to the women who knit for the newborns at the hospital.

The woman pulls up in front of the house and comes to the door.

"Hello, I'm Martha. I understand you have some yarn for me to pick up?"

"Oh yes, thanks for coming. I can't fit it all in my car with my son's car seat or I would have come by with it."

"Oh." Martha is perplexed. Normal amounts of yarn wouldn't take up much space. I lead her back out to the yard, to the pile of garbage bags next to the gate.

"Here you go." I smile as she just looks and looks.

"This is yarn?"

"Yeah, it's all new. I just realized I wasn't a knitter after all." Actually, I'm not a lot of the things I once was.

"Wow, okay. Well, thank you! We'll make good use of it."

I help her load it up, one bag after another, stuffed with my shopping mania and big ideas. As she drives away, I feel the weight of a thousand unfinished projects slide from my back. What a relief. Another small miracle—relief.

I asked Dad about his miracle. He knew I would never have made it through the telling of the story of his supplements back when he started me on them at the Cardston house. So he hadn't told me much about his miracle back then. Now he gave the story to me in pieces, bit by bit, a hint here, a laugh there. I didn't truly put the pieces together until I read a newspaper article. It was a story about me and Joe and Mom and our madness. The reporter put the story in order. As miracles go, it was a good one.

Dad, a brilliant, well-educated man with a string of successful businesses, had been brought down. His humble job, maintaining church buildings, carpets and toilets and drinking fountains, let him slouch and fidget and reckon, seeking the solution to a problem unlike any engineering problem he'd ever tackled at our kitchen table. It was the problem that had wrecked our lives.

Like many people, he found his answer in a church. But not in prayer. Instead, it was in a hallway, where he met David Hardy.

David was a soft-spoken humble man, who wore white button-down shirts and grey polyester slacks, who combed his hair to the side and stuck it down firmly around the ears. He had started out as a high school biology teacher and had moved on, for the last twenty years, working his own business as a pig-feed salesman and formulator.

And Dad, seeing this man, so composed, so humble and kind, found it in himself to drag out the family laundry bag and air it in the hallway. After all those years of denial, he let the truth out all at once. The stench must have made David's eyes water. He smelled the part about Mom, dead and cold in the ground. He sniffed the part about me, crazed and drugged and sitting with a full bladder playing solitaire on the couch because the devil was in the bathroom mirror and Dana was not home yet to escort me to the toilet. And he choked when Joe's story wafted up and bit his nostrils, and he knew this good boy was ill and violent and that he would never have a normal life, let alone happiness. David wept for Dad and all of Dad's dirty laundry, and then he said the most remarkable thing.

"That boy sounds like a pig with ear-and-tail-biting syndrome."

I can only imagine what I might have said if a man had told me my son had a sickness unique to pigs. Dad asked how David treated it. David said he knew a good ratio of trace minerals and major minerals that helped calm the pigs. They decided to try it out on me and Joe.

I had tried the first version before Christmas, before the dining room table and the hospital, before Dana's ring went missing. No help. Not for me and not for Joe. We slept better for a while, but sanity eluded us.

Dad and David didn't give up. They kept tweaking. They searched the market for human-grade supplements that would match David's pig-feed formulation. And when Dad found the missing piece, he was so certain. We both were.

He was certain it would work, and I was just as certain it wouldn't. I played along. For Dad's sake. He was so desperate, so guilty about Mom, so needy. He needed to at least try to save me. So I let him try. I didn't have anything to lose.

The miracle of the discovery was not lost on us. My strength came back. By summertime I was hiking and riding my bike. I put my handicapped parking placard away for good. I still wavered between good and bad days, but I marvelled at the changes in my health and mourned for the lost years.

I was clear and predictable. I was off all my psychotropic drugs. No lithium, no Prozac, no Paxil, no Tegretol, no Haldol, no Rivotril, no Ativan, no Cogentin, no Epival. And none of the others, the nameless drugs slipped into me in needles and during psych ward stays. None of those given to me in trial and error, one experimental combination after another, the doctors waiting to see what good—or what damage—the latest experiment might do, never having a clue as to what outcome to expect until they saw it. And now this. No prescriptions. No wild outcomes. Nothing but a natural food supplement.

Discovering my new life took patience. The photo album was full of pictures of me on vacation in places I had never been: Las Vegas, Vancouver, Seattle, Utah. Dana sat and flipped the pages and told me about my life during the previous three years when I had been here in body, but not in soul and seldom enough in mind.

Adjusting to the quiet in my head took practice, and sometimes I missed the excitement, the high of my mania. Sometimes normal was boring.

"What are you doing?" Dana has joined me on the lawn. I'm picking at the grass.

"I'm boring."

"Bored?"

"No, boring. I miss the creativity. I'm boring."

"I like you boring."

I think of the decidedly un-boring moments I've given him. I can see why he'd positively adore boring. But . . .

"Do you like me? I struggled all these years to come back, and now I'm here and I don't like myself."

"It'll come, babe. You'll find your balance."

He likes me boring. Suddenly it hits me—hard. A new phase of my wellness. I stop thinking about me and think about Dana. He has been here all along, living through my madness. I see me through his point of view. I have hurt him, shamed him, scared him.

"I'm so sorry, Dana, for the pain, for all the things that I did and said to hurt you."

"I know." He kisses me. "I love you. I thought I would just be with you until you died. I was sure you would die. I'm so glad you are alive and with me. It's still Love Only."

From Dana's point of view I could give it up, the creativity. The ideas, music, and voices did not improve me. The mania was not brilliance. I would find my balance. I would stay boring. He loved me.

But I found I did not have to give up creativity after all. I began to write about it all, about Dana and my mom and all the pain and all the love. I wrote about coming to know my dad, loving him, my prayerful, inspired hero. The men who saved my life. My heroes. There was healing in my writing. Then Dad introduced me to another way to heal.

"You need to talk about it, Autumn. We're having a meeting in the basement of David's home. A bunch of people want to meet you and hear your story."

I was mortified. "No. I don't want to talk about it, Dad. It's too embarrassing. It's too hard to keep bringing it up. I'm still trying to get past it. Don't make me wallow in it."

"If you won't talk, then who will? How will anyone get help if they can't hear about what you used to be like?"

"That's just my point. I don't want to be the formerly crazy person. I just want to be who I am now. Dredging up all that crap would be like getting naked in public. I don't need the embarrassment."

"You go home and pray about this and then tell me what you're going to do. I think you should talk."

I was grateful to Dad and thankful to David and I wanted to help other people, I really did, but talking meant opening myself up to public scrutiny and possibly even mockery. Now that I could see my illness from the other side, there was a lot of humiliation in it. Dad was asking me to relive the depths of it—not in private, not in a hospital assessment room, but in a packed basement filled with strangers.

Could I fix other people with my story, when I didn't even know how it would end? How could I help strangers when my own home was filled with strangers? I didn't know my family yet. Yet they had lived my story with me. They were a part of my story. How could I subject them to the telling of it?

36

Little Boy Blue, come blow your horn,
The sheep's in the meadow, the cow's in the corn.
Where's Little Boy Blue? I don't hear a peep . . .
Oh, he's under the haystack fast asleep.

My boy with no refuge, no horn, and no hay.
My little boy, with no place to stay.
He's sad and he's lonely, there's no hand to hold.
He's raising himself till he turns three years old.

James. Little Boy Blue, I called him. He was so serious.

No more daycare for my son. I was newly reformed, on the road to a lifetime of recovery. I had stopped taking the last drug, Epival. I was ready. Ready for my second chance at motherhood. I was calm and clear. Ready.

I was also busy. I was on a quest to understand where I had been. I wanted to know what the aftermath of my drug use would be. I had to conquer the issues of addiction and dependence. I was curious about family abuse patterns. I wanted to learn all there was to know about herbal remedies, alternative methods for coping with stress, and natural healing. Vitamins and minerals and natural therapies. One such therapy was saving my life. It was important. It was good. I had other good things in my life. I could read now. I had time. I did read.

James. He spent his days hanging out near me, behind me, underfoot. He talked nonstop. His questions were unrelenting. He made up endless stories about his guts and brain and lungs. He begged me to read from his favourite books, all of them about nature and animals and human anatomy. But he didn't stop talking long enough to listen when I read to him. He jabbered over my reading, on and on about what his body was doing. Talk-talk-talk-talk-talk. I had a hard time listening. I had a hard time reading. All that talking.

James. He loved information, books, pamphlets, anything with pictures that made him think he could decipher the meaning of the words on the page. He took in countless hours of Discovery Channel. He tried to understand his world, and what he couldn't understand he would fill in with brilliant three-year-old theories and ideas that he took for truth. And he had theories about everything. Some kids obsess over dinosaurs. James obsessed over anatomy and physiology and the mechanics of life.

"How does my blood grab the oxygen? How, Mom? There are no fingers on this red blood cell. The picture doesn't have any fingers. See? See? How does it, Mom? How does it grab the oxygen?"

"I don't know."

"Oh, it must have the sticky stuff, like on the scab, the gluey stuff that makes it stick together. That must stick the oxygen, Mom. Right, Mom? Right, Mom?"

"Mmmhmmm."

Birds, flowers, the atmosphere, trees, leaves, dirt, worms, his body, my body, metal, glass, the television, the VCR, the toaster—he had to know how everything worked. It was a whole lot of talking.

It didn't bother me, exactly. I seldom heard him except as background chatter.

James. Day in and day out.

Me. Conjuring up my own theories and plans for healing in my own head.

James in my ears. Me in my head.

"Mom, did you know that I have a heart? It's a muscle that moves my blood around, and I can feel it go pump pump pump pump pump pump pump . . ." James is standing by my left leg while I am doing a sink of dishes. I have just finished reading a document about Haldol poisoning.

"Mmmhmmm." Those awful drugs.

"And my blood takes the air from my lungs and grabs out the oxygen and puts it in my brain and my liver and my pancreas so I can live."

"Wow, mmmhmmm." I slop another dirty pot into the warm soapy water. I'm thinking about the long-term storage of drugs in fat tissue.

"And then my bum makes the poop come out so I don't get full of all of my food."

"Mmmhmm." I remember the load of laundry I left in the washer overnight. I go to see if it is too stinky to put in the dryer. James follows after me, rambling on. Something about poop and pee and oxygen.

"I'm worried about James."

"Why?" Dana is removing his watch and emptying the gum wrappers and loose change from his work pants.

"He's not normal." I am sitting on the end of the bed.

"What are you talking about?"

"He's not normal. This morning I asked him to come to the breakfast table and eat and he wouldn't, so I went over to get him and he hit the floor."

"Hit the floor?"

"Yeah, as if he ducked to avoid me. I wasn't going to hit him. It was just about cereal. I wasn't going to hit him."

"He's really been tossed around by this thing, hasn't he?" Dana steps out of his work pants.

"I know he has, but I don't even know where to begin fixing it."

Dana nods and slides out of his shirt.

"It's just so disturbing. He ducks when I move toward him, but he won't leave me alone for five seconds. This kid will talk for an hour straight and never give up. He just follows me around rattling off facts from Discovery Channel and that dumb human body picture book that we got him."

Dana stuffs his clothes in the hamper.

"He doesn't even look at me. He just follows me around and stares at the wall and tries to occupy my head with this stuff. I can't think any of my own thoughts without him trying to take over my head space."

Dana pulls on a pair of shorts and stands in front of me. "Have you tried looking at him?"

We are face to face. I divert my gaze to the hamper.

"What does that have to do with—"

He takes me by the shoulder and turns me to face him. Eye to eye. His eyes are kind and blue. But intense. He knows something about me that I need to know. I can see it's something I don't want to know.

"Just look at him."

Oh no. What does James know that I don't?

"Hey, Jimbo, it's time for breakfast." James comes in from his bedroom with a heap of wind-up construction toys clutched to his narrow toddler chest. I have a couple of bowls of cold cereal waiting for us and another article about benzodiazepine addiction to review.

"It's a busy morning, kiddo, so hop up and get eating." He doesn't move toward the table. He goes to the slate floor in front of the fireplace and starts setting up his construction site.

"C'mon, James. The cereal's getting soggy, get up here now."

I get off my chair and walk over to get him. He ducks away.

He ducks. Doesn't say no or have a fit and demand to play with his backhoes and ploughs. He just ducks.

I leave him to play and go back to the table. I pick up my article. I begin to read. He comes to me. *Now that I am occupied, he comes to me?*

"Mom, Mom, did you know that dogs and cats and elephants are like us but snakes aren't? Snakes don't have babies that are alive—well, they are alive, but they're in eggs like chickens so they don't breathe air and neither do baby alligators, and the eggs are in the dirt except for chickens 'cause they have nests, not dirt piles . . ."

"Mmmhmm."

Ignoring him has become so automatic. I catch myself. *Just look at him.* I set down my paper and turn in my chair to face James. Little James. He is looking at the seat cover on his chair. He is rambling on at full speed. " . . .when they come out they get air and it is just like when human babies get born because the air supply stops from the mom and they have to breathe with lungs like mine . . ."

He puts his chubby hand to his chest and thumps it.

"I have lungs, too," I say, leaning down to him.

He meets my gaze. He looks back at the chair. He looks back at me as if to see if I'm still there.

"What do your lungs do?" I ask.

He is flustered. He stammers, "My lungs bring the air so the blood can grab it . . . I'm hungry."

He clambers into his chair to eat, and we have a quiet breakfast. He eats. I just look at him, my James.

I look at him all morning. And every day from then on. Now that I see him, I want to discover all there is to know about this mystery that is my boy. His hair is still baby-fine. His face is pale and soft and dimpled in the chin and on his cheeks. He has my eyes, wide and blue and almond shaped. His smile is full of ground-down baby teeth, ultra-white and clean.

He is overly concerned with tooth brushing. He is meticulous about his hands never being sticky or stinky, although there is always a trace of breakfast or lunch on his cheeks and shirt collar. He is smart and tall and fiercely independent, yet he is still unable to use the toilet or button his shirt or cut with scissors. He cries easily and is quick to fly into rages when things don't go his way. He can sit for hours without being entertained, but he never leaves my side.

Every time he calls my name from that day on, I answer with a word instead of a grunt. And I look into his eyes. He shies away from that. I see he is threatened by me when I look at him. And I know at last what I have done, what Dana knows but never told me, what James remembers but I do not.

I am so, so sad. This blond fluffy-haired little boy has done everything he could think of to be a part of my world these last years. He has spent countless days at my bedside, chewing on apples and watching documentaries and educational TV. Careful not to disturb me. Hoping that, in my lethargy, I would let him be near me. Yet fearful of the nearness to the sleeping lioness, hoping I would never look him in the eye, for that was to risk a smack or a rant of verbal abuse.

Three years of my absenteeism while he was at my very side. Three years of his wondering if he could ever be interesting enough or valiant enough or good enough or bad enough to catch my gaze without catching the back of my hand.

Oh, Little Boy Blue, I am so, so sorry.

37

Just when it seemed I had my family back, Dad decided it was time to start helping other families. At first Dad thought he'd made a real discovery. He and David would share it with doctors who would, of course, accept it and want to use it, and they would help so many more people than Dad could ever reach. Then Mom's death would not be in vain, and people would know that they didn't have to die the way she died. *Not so simple.*

Real discoveries are made by scientists, not by a couple of small town laymen from southern Alberta.

"Hey, Autumn." Dad is calling. "I had an interesting chat with the good Dr. Taylor today." Dr. Taylor is indeed good. I remember him from Mom's funeral, a well-respected, kind man with a sincere desire to help our family in our time of need.

"Oh, really? What did you chat about?"

"Well, I took Barb in with the baby, and during the appointment I brought up the minerals and how well you and Joe were doing. I asked him if he'd like to try the supplement on any of his patients because, you know, it's a small town and we all know who's suffering out there. Then he puts down his pen and looks right at me and tells me I shouldn't be doing it. I shouldn't even be talking about it."

"What?"

"Yeah, he says I am practicing illegal medicine and I could be thrown in jail for it."

"Practicing medicine?" *Not exactly.*

"Yeah, ha, more like practicing nutrition." Dad laughs, but not whole-heartedly.

This was the first time a doctor had told Dad to stop what he was doing, but it most certainly wouldn't be the last. Rejection after rejection, mockery and rolling eyes, legs and arms crossed and heads shaking. No.

No, Tony, this is no discovery.

No, Tony, your kids are just in remission.

No, Tony, you have nothing here, *nothing.*

But you ought to be careful, Tony.

The repeated rejection and the implied threat of jail led Dad to make another kind of call. He called the College of Physicians and Surgeons just to be sure he wasn't crossing a line.

"You called them? What if they decide to investigate you?" I am gripping the phone and picturing Dad in the back of a paddy wagon with bars on the windows and a siren on top, wailing for the neighbourhood to come and see. And Dad's kids, all the little ones jumping up and down on the lawn and wailing louder than the siren, *Please bring our daddy back, he's not practicing medicine!*

"Don't worry, I told them everything and they said I can talk about vitamins and minerals as much as I want. And I can talk about mental illness, too, as long as I am not pretending to be a doctor. I have to make it clear that I am a layman."

"Oh, good. So there's no trouble then." The sirens stop and my heart slows to normal.

"Anyway, I'm definitely not a doctor. I wouldn't call myself one of them if they begged me. Seriously, Autumn, I have never seen so many closed-minded people."

"How can they be so closed-minded and in charge of health care?" I ask.

"Well, that's just it. David says they aren't in charge of anything. Doctors only know what they are told. Scientists are the real thinkers. We have been knocking on the wrong doors."

It was evident that no one in medical practice was interested in Dad and David's claim of discovery. They were laymen challenging medicine with pigpen logic. Laymen claiming to know something the psychiatrists didn't know. Laymen asking for change in a multi-billion-dollar industry, while their discovery was still less than a year old. If the medical world wouldn't take them seriously, maybe the people who were actually suffering would be willing to listen and document their own responses to the supplement. Maybe then they could get a real thinker to pay attention.

We are coming up on the third anniversary of Mom's suicide, and Dad wants to do something to be sure her death was not in vain.

"Silence kills, Autumn. We can't be silent about this. We can't hide what we know. People need to know this. There are people dying because no one will talk about it. We need to talk." Dad will no longer keep secrets. He will not sweep under a carpet the ugly truth about where we have been. He wants to make it right for Mom. In memory of Mom.

Dad and David start Truehope, a company for supporting people with bipolar disorders, chronic depression, and the like. And I find that I want to speak after all. I want to give hope to others.

The room, a grungy basement conference hall in a cheap northside hotel, is dotted with about fifty earnest faces. Dad starts by sharing the family story. David talks about the discovery of the supplement. I am to share my personal success with it.

". . . and I have been well for over eight months now—with no medication," I conclude with great satisfaction.

I expect applause. There is none.

"Who do you think you are?" a woman at the back of the room wants to know. She gets to her feet and lectures me on the danger of offering false hope. She says it is wrong. She says I have no right to declare that I am well when I am clearly only in an average remission of symptoms. The woman says we are fakes and frauds, trying to take advantage of the poor and helpless, the mentally ill. She goes on and on.

I can see it in her. She is me as I once was, and my mother before me. She is the centre of her universe. I try not to feel offended by her attack. I know she has said the same things to her doctors and psychiatrists. I know she has said the same things to everybody. I know her better than she would ever guess. But still . . .

I didn't want to speak any more. I couldn't sell my mother and her death. I couldn't sell my illness and my recovery. Not to people like her. I went home discouraged. And I know Dad was discouraged, too.

But Dad kept calling me to ask me to speak, and I kept showing up. How could I refuse? I owed him my life. I owed Mom something, too. Dad and David booked halls and meeting rooms. We spoke in basements of homes and in stinky community centres with terrible acoustics and rickety orange stackable chairs.

"If it helps just—"

"I know, Dad. If we help just one person avoid Mom's suffering, then it's worth it."

"That's right."

"But I hate talking about my illness, Dad."

I didn't tell him how truly tough it was. I didn't tell him it made me vomit. But I kept going, and in spite of the continued opposition from the medical community the venues changed. We were bolder. We spoke in hospital auditoriums and college classrooms. The press began to call. The effort was worth it. The normals were beginning to believe me.

A cure for mental illness? A natural supplement conforming to the principles David Hardy had learned in formulating pig feed? It seemed reasonable to all of us. David and Dad had simply applied the same principles to formulating a supplement for humans. A supplement made, not of pig feed, and certainly not derived from pigs, but of human-grade vitamins and minerals combined in a safe manufacturing process.

The press leapt on it. They leapt ahead of it, too, to absurd conclusions and preposterous claims. The supplement became a "pig pill." A magic pig pill that, depending on the press slant, either cured mental illness in pigs and could therefore cure mentally ill humans, too. Or a pig pill that was used simply to scam the mentally ill.

The very idea of a miracle pig pill made people giddy. People wanted studies. Dad and David wanted studies.

I didn't need a study. I knew. The supplement alleviated my bipolar symptoms. And it allowed me to get off the cocktails of less-than-miraculous drugs. Which was fine by me. I didn't believe in magic cures;

I just wanted a cure that made sense. One with limitations and a viable explanation. There was only one way to find the limits of Dad and David's supplement. I would have to go off it and see. But . . .

Too bad. Going off the supplement was one thing I told myself I would never do, no matter how much it might further the advance of science and medicine. At least not voluntarily. But then I got a sinus infection. I went to the doctor and he prescribed antibiotics. The antibiotics killed the bacteria in my gut as well as the stuff in my sinuses. I got diarrhea. But that's not all.

I began to slip back into that agitation that I knew as the first stage of my mania. I was so afraid. Afraid my miracle was at an end. My doctor was shocked. He could see it, too, in the pacing, the tapping, forms of repetitious behaviour that were edging me closer to flapping.

He studied my charts and found his answer. The antibiotics had killed the bacteria I needed to digest my food, causing diarrhea that flushed the supplement out of my system before I could absorb it.

He told me to triple my supplements and come back in four days. By the end of the week I was one of the normals again. I realized now how fragile my condition was and how necessary the supplements were. Call them magic in the press, if you like. Or call them pig pills. Either way, I had to have a sure supply of them.

Knowing I needed them and could not be stable without them gave me courage to speak out in other ways. There was a movement, a rebellion, brewing in Canada. The bureaucratic body responsible for health issues, Health Canada, was implementing new regulations that exerted tight control over health food stores, the importation of natural health products from the United States, where our supplement was made, and the manufacture of natural supplements within Canada.

"If they succeed with this," Dad told me, "you will not have access to the minerals any more. All of it will have to be regulated as pharmaceutical drugs, and it will cost millions in research and take years to get back on the market. Canada will be like Australia, with no access to natural stuff." He was concerned, and I was fearful that the supplement could be pulled off the market, and I would have to go back to being sick. Angela and Sunni and I vowed to give the fight our best efforts, so that this doesn't happen.

There were community gatherings and town hall meetings, petition drives, and radio talk shows demanding that natural foods not be treated the same as drugs. I spoke, Dad spoke, David spoke, Sunni gathered petitions, Angela arranged meeting halls. We joined forces with health freedom groups all across the country, and millions of Canadians stood up and demanded change. They wanted health freedom, too.

We knew we'd been a part of something significant when Minister of Health Alan Rock called for change himself and set up a committee to respond to the petitions. I felt safer. When Mr. Rock accepted the fifty-three recommendations of the committee and set up a transition team to expand and clarify them, I felt victorious. Mr. Rock said the recommendations were as good as law, that we would soon see Canadian legislation change.

Sections 3.1 and 3.2 and Schedule A of the Food and Drug Act would be abolished. These sections were crucial to me because the three of them together made it illegal for me to claim that the supplement changed my illness. Under law, only pharmaceutical drugs could claim to help the symptoms of any disease listed in Schedule A, and bipolar was one of them. Now I felt secure. Finally. The government was changing law to allow free access to supplements that worked. Canadians were achieving true health freedom.

The law didn't change right away, however. The Liberal government did some shuffling in the ranks and responsibilities of the top cabinet ministers. I should have been afraid. I should have been suspicious. But I wasn't. Because my dad was part-owner of the company that supplied the supplement, I felt confident that I would always have first access to the supply that Truehope imported from the United States. In fact, I felt confident enough to want another baby.

I tried to get pregnant for three years, but without success. I went for fertility testing. The gynecologist said I wasn't ovulating. I tried hormone therapy, but that sent my moods spiralling out of control. Dana and I chose my sanity over a baby. We gave up.

As the heavy snowfall of 1999 melted into a damp and mouldy spring, I became sick. So sick that I was forced to see the doctor. Autoimmunity, he called it. He wanted to prescribe a steroid known to cause mood disorder in people who are predisposed to that type of illness. For me, predisposed wasn't the word for it.

"I can't. I can't take that drug."

"Then there is nothing else I can offer you."

"I'd rather be crippled than crazy again. This will pass. Crazy might not."

My condition worsened, however, and I became bedridden. I could only rise to drag my legs to the bathroom.

There are always those who break the rules, those who claim magic cures and unsubstantiated forms of healing. Those who prey on the hopeless, the desperately ill. They offer easy answers and nonsense potions. Because of this, I never trusted the people I lumped together in my mind as "the alternative types."

But when I could not endure the raised hot skin any more, I gave in to a friend's prompting and called a homeopath who specialized in natural remedies. *And maybe a bit of magic?*

Dr. Sandhar was very friendly. He was an old man with a turban and a thin see-through beard that reached to his navel. I sat across from him as he asked me for a summary of my medical history. He chuckled as the story went on and on and on. He nodded and put up his hand: *Okay, okay, enough of this history. I get it, I get it.*

"The drugs have hurt your organs. Give me three months. We will have you fixed up. Okay?" He scribbled on a note pad and tore off the sheet.

"Okay. Thank you." I reached for the prescription of tinctures and a pamphlet on diet. *Three months?*

"You have more questions?"

"Three months?"

"Yes, yes."

Another thing that's always on my mind. "I don't ovulate."

"Oh, well." He laughed, tossing his head back and ruffling his beard.

"Do not worry. If you follow this protocol, you will have as many babies as you want. Okay? As many as you want."

Ridiculous. Years of infertility and he's going to fix the whole thing in a few weeks with some drops and a yeast-free diet?

Insane. As insane as pig pills. Yes, yes, indeed.

I went home and did everything he said.

38

Not having babies made me different from my mother. And now, in her absence, that broke my heart. I needed her. Not the sick woman who drowned in the thick exhaust of her final fury; not her. I needed the mother I once knew in the garden, with wisdom, patience, and calm. I needed her to tell me I was all right, that I was acceptable to her.

I wrote poetry and journal entries of every kind, to find myself, to sort out what was me and what was Mom. Which parts would stay and which would go as the illness left my body, as a new strength filled it. I wrote to discover myself. It was then, during this period of self-discovery, that I realized I was missing pieces, not just memories taken by the drugs. I was missing entire chapters, like a book slammed closed on my fingers. I wanted the whole story. And I knew who could give it to me.

My hands are deep in warm dishwater. Comfortable outside, torn inside. I am tired of memories void of emotion and feeling. All the smells, the tastes, all the senses are sucked from them. They are sketched out in charcoal, cropped close around the edges, empty, shallow. I want to feel my life, *all of it.*

"Give me the rest of it."

No. My Girl is apprehensive.

"I want it. I want it all. Full colour. Full frame. It's my life. I'll never be whole without the whole truth."

It's too much.

"I'm better now, I'm grown. I can handle it. You have to show me. It's mine."

You don't want to feel this.

But I do.

My Girl gives it all up: a cyclone of memories both sweet and excruciating. I am blown over by the wind, the snap and flap of filth on the clothesline of my mind. Each sheet is a moment in time My Girl had tucked and folded away in a closet. Each one is now wide open, flying and whipping in the wind.

I don't just see the separate moments now. I feel them, as though for the first time. The pain, the confusion, the terror. Gordy, his face, his lips. The teen girl, her fists, and Mom's battered eyes. And Grandpa, his secret kept by Mom. And Mom again. At the river, in the shower, in the van, in the mortuary.

And my own fists. I see my own fists, and my little boy's eyes, confusion in his face, tears on his cheeks. I see myself throwing away my medication and taking James on the bus, far away. I see Shawna driving. Then we are at her house, and I am drunk with mania; glue and paint, wood and cloth, dried flowers and ceramic pieces are scattered over her table, and James is motherless, an orphan to a manic crafting episode, and Shawna is tired, and I am embarrassed. I see me, struggling to diaper my boy. He is laughing and I am furious. And then, and then—I see the dam burst and the mania becomes flapping and the flapping becomes slapping and I am slapping my baby and screaming and Shawna is there and her husband is holding James and I am in the hospital and then I'm home again. And Dana is saying, "I love you, but if you ever, ever go off your medication again, I will take my son and go and you will never see us. You will not be that kind of a mother to my child."

I have to accept that I have not just been a victim; I have been a perpetrator, too. I wail and vomit in the sink. I crouch on the floor and howl and writhe, and I think that I might die in this moment. The pain. Too much. It's too much for me. But not for Him. And I feel Him near.

Then I see them all for what they are. Every perpetrator in my life. They are people like me, the broken and the lost. Like me. He loved them, too, each in his time, each in his own pain, each in his own ashes. He loved them. He loved them, so I can't hate them either. At the moment that I feel the pain, face it fully and feel theirs, too, I start on my path to forgiveness.

I am forgiven when I forgive them. He forgave them—and me. He kept His promise and declared the victory—*liberty to the captives*. And I am freed. Bound no more in illness, in torment, in pain, in anger, in hatred. *Free*.

On that day in the kitchen, the day My Girl and I become one again, each moment on that clothesline in my mind is washed clean and hung out again. *I have found me, Dad, I found me, and I am so blessed.*

Being my mother no longer made me cringe. Now being her, knowing her, and all of me, made me whole. And I was ready to embrace my new identity. After all, Mom and I always needed to be needed. And I found the most needful souls in my community. I was one of them; not cured but recovering. I knew the illness from the inside. I could use the words that other people could never get away with.

There were always people seeking Truehope. Many of them found it on my green couch. Not with the Bible, as I did. Not with My Girl, as I did. Not with a vision like mine. But with me, Autumn, in open, honest conversation. They tested me, and found I was one of them. Some decided Truehope wasn't for them. But least they knew they had a choice.

Beatrice shows up with her luggage, her coat and hat and sneakers, her favourite box of tea, and her electric kettle. She is a grandma, a Mrs. Claus type, and she is moving out of her home. Today she woke up knowing that her faithful husband of forty-three years is a loser—in fact, a killer. She knows me from my Truehope presentations and will not leave. So . . .

"Beatrice, please, come in," I tell her. She shakes and fumbles as she comes through the door. And then without a word or warning, she wails. She's doing the ugly cry in short dramatic bursts, and I'm suspicious.

I hold her puffy body and touch her frazzled hair and say, "Come in, let's sit you down."

"I need you to help me." Her voice is soft and the cry is already forgotten.

"I know. I'm glad you came."

"I can't live with him any more."

"What happened?"

"He's a killer." There's the word. I know the rest of the game. She puts the back of her hand to her forehead, like Scarlet O'Hara, about to faint.

"Beatrice, this man has been with you through years and years of illness. You are on the edge of getting well. But you've spent thirty years on the drugs, and a lot of habits have developed. You need to do your part now. Fight for this. Just give it a few more weeks, fight for this chance at a real life."

"I can't."

"Do you want it?"

"I want to be well, but I'm weak, and he is expecting so much from me. He says now that I'm awake all day instead of drugged and sleeping, I ought to take care of the house a little. He fired the housekeeper."

"Oh." I picture myself crawling up the stairs, too weak to help Mom Stringam with dinner. *So very seriously tired.* "Are you angry?"

"I just need someone to take care of me. I need someone to bring me food in my bed."

"You can't have it both ways. If you are well, you need to start acting well and doing normal things."

"I served him for years before I got sick. Years. And now he expects me to mop the floor again?" Her voice is changing from soft to gruff and not so grandma-like.

"Are you sick?"

"No."

"Are you drugged?"

"No."

"Beatrice, you have to choose. I know it's tough to take on responsibility. Everyone wants to stay in bed and watch television sometimes. Normal people don't stay in bed. You have to choose to get up. No one said getting normal would be easy. Normal people work."

"I don't want to hurt you, you know."

"What?"

She's turning it on, playing the game. She's going to do whatever it takes to be admitted and certified in a psych ward. There they bring the food and do your laundry. You don't have to be a mom. You don't have to be a wife. You can be a sick person. *Whatever it takes.* In her case, to show her husband that he isn't the boss of her. She snarls and sneers and leans in to my face. I smell her acrid breath and I am not moved.

"I don't want to hurt you. But I can see it. Your face, your blood. Oh please, don't let me hurt you, don't let me do it." She's not begging, she's threatening, and her eyes are wide and devious.

"Cut the crap."

"What?" Her face relaxes at once.

"I played that game, Bea. I did it, too, and I know the rules. Cut the crap and settle down. If you want to go to bed and watch television for the rest of your life, then say so, and I'll take you to the hospital. But you won't do it here. And you and I both know you don't have to any more." *You're busted.*

She gives me a knowing smirk. "I'm just so mad at him."

Ahh, now the truth.

"You have to learn how to work it out. You have to undo the thirty years of sickness. You have to redo the way you live with each other. You have to negotiate."

"Just let me stay here for a week or so, and then he'll want me back."

"No. You can get room service in a hotel or a hospital or you can go home and face your past."

She makes her decision. She apologizes for the death threat. *No problem, Bea. Who am I to judge you for being manipulative or ill?* She asks me to drive her to the hospital.

I tell her I will. She requests the back seat and the child lock. *No problem. I know how it works.*

She howls in the hallway. They put her and me into an isolation room, thinking I am her daughter.

"Are you sure you want this?"

"Yeah." She is sitting on the edge of the bed, talking normally.

"They'll put you on drugs again."

"It's easier that way." Bea stretches and yawns.

"I think it's a mistake."

"It's my life." She shrugs. *She's right. Absolutely.*

The doctor walks in, and Bea goes evil. Bea goes tyrannical, Bea goes coy. Bea flirts. I sit in the corner and cry a little and shake my head. I do not like this picture. They fill out the papers and put on the multicoloured bracelet.

The doctor is satisfied. He asks me into the hall. I tell him I'm not a blood relation, just a casual friend, but he isn't put off by that. He's perfectly willing to discuss her case.

"She's really out there, eh?" Not like us normals, eh? I wipe my face. I am sad that she chose the illness.

"We'll load her up," he says. "Get her some sleep. We get these kinds in all the time."

"What's her prognosis?" *One normal to another.*

"Oh, y'know. It's bipolar. You never get over that."

"Yeah. I guess not." He doesn't know I am more like her than like him, and I won't tell him otherwise. Instead I ask, "Have you heard about that Truehope program?"

"Oh, the vitamin thing. Yeah, I saw it in the press." He laughs. I laugh with him.

"What do you think? Is it worth trying?"

"Are you kidding? Your friend is way beyond vitamins. It's a scam, anyway."

"Really? I heard it worked."

"Well, I don't believe it. If it worked, we'd be using it here." He smiles, one normal to another, taps his clipboard, and walks away.

And I walk away, back into my normal life. I leave Bea in the hospital. I just walk away. Past her door, pushing through the double fire doors, down the emergency hall, and out the automatic sliding door. It slides and bumps and I step out into the sunshine. And I remember the moment I left Mom in the shower with her devious kitten smirk, and I feel the guilt wash over me.

How I wish I could have saved my mother, and Beatrice, this soft grandma, someone's wife, someone else's mom. I want to shout out. I want to tell the world about my recovery and save everyone else the thirty years that Bea has spent in pain.

Meanwhile, there are grumbles of trouble for Dad and for David. I hear snippets about letters and phone calls and trips to Ottawa. Dad and Dana are protecting me, shielding me, saving me from the stress of it all, but I hear enough to know. Enough to know that I want no part in the drama, and that I want it to end soon, so we can just get on with helping other people like me. Like Mom, like Bea.

39

Another garden, another prairie. We're twelve hours north of my mother's prairie garden on the acreage. I am twenty-nine and strong and healthy and I am not alone. I hear James tromping up the driveway and pushing through the gate. I look up from my place on my knees in the soil to see him as he comes around the corner. He is tall. His broad shoulders and thick wrists remind me of Dana's. He is much larger than other children his age. He's healthy, and smart, and he has a sense of humour that rivals any adult's wit. He is almost nine.

"Mom, can I ride my bike to the park? Brady and I want to fly our jet planes." James has hopped up onto the broad warm deck. His entire hobby kit is stuffed under his arm. Foam wings, wires, and the top of an air pump are protruding every which way.

"Okay, just be sure to get back for supper."

"Great, um, do you know where my helmet is?"

"It's in the shed." He pops in and back out at once.

"I can't find it."

I push up from my knees and go to him. I duck into the shed and grab the helmet from the tangled mess of tires and wires and outdoor play stuff.

"It's in the garden shed, right where you left it." I trade him the helmet for a kiss. He frees a hand and takes it, then kisses me back.

"Thanks, Mom."

"Okay, have fun."

He is off. I return to my garden plot. He does not duck from me now.

When our eyes meet, there is understanding without fear.

The garden shed—it was one of the first reasons I fell in love with this house. It was built to match the home exterior, with clean white siding and gray shingles, and a window bordered in evergreen paint. It's a hiding place for messy stuff: my bags of potting soil and my stacks of terra cotta pots and planters. Now, in June, it is nearly empty because the planters have been filled and brought out to brighten the stairs and walkways of our luscious green corner lot. It's a good space for James to store his bike and scooter and all of his playthings, so the deck can be kept safe for Samantha.

Samantha. Where is she?

I turn on my knees in the dirt to spot her toddling in the shade, shuffling through a bed of white blossoms, a dusting of fragrant snow from the apple tree.

"Do you want to come help me, baby? Mommy is pulling weeds. If you want to put them in the bucket, that would be so nice."

She runs to me, faster than her little legs can carry her, and stumbles in the grass. She lands on her hands in the dirt. Her blonde fluff of fine hair is tossed into her eyes. Before I can get to her, she is on her feet again, smiling and jabbering.

" 'At's okay."

"Okay? Do you want the bucket?"

She steps through the soil to reach me, and I trade a bucket for a wet kiss. Her wide blue eyes are deep and knowing. Samantha is an old soul in a baby girl's body. She is the crowning jewel in my garden, the first testament to me that there is a chance of life after mental illness.

I remember the day she was born.

I laboured for hours with her, my eyes closed, singing to myself, moaning and breathing, and tormented with pain. I thought it would never end—and then suddenly, she came.

"Look, hon, open your eyes."

"I can't."

"Look. You have to open your eyes."

I opened my eyes, first to the sight of Dana, tears streaming down his face, and the window behind him filled with the morning sun. It was Christmas Eve morning, heralding the dawn of our own miracle baby with a sky of fuchsia and mauve and gold.

Dana put her on my chest, tiny and strong and loud. Samantha. A gift. *The gift.* The fulfillment of God's promise to bring, in trade for my sorrow and my weakness, Samantha.

Now with the spring breeze in my ponytail and my knees damp in the moist black soil, I am her mother. I am in my own prairie garden, guarded by a tall fence and tucked in the shade of old trees. Samantha is my little helper, and my hips are aching. Another blessing has come our way; another baby will be born two months from now. I reach beyond my round belly to grab the last of the thistle that has sprung up among my potato plants. My gloves protect my fingernails, since they are long now and no longer bitten-down like Mom's.

Not like Mom's. I am suddenly overcome with emotion for this moment, in my garden, like a mirror image of my mother's garden but with a future that will never mirror hers. My tears water the soil.

"Thank you," I whisper from my knees. "Thank you for the sun and the wind and my baby girl. Thank you for my dad, my Dana, and my James. Thank you for all of this."

40

My story should have ended there, in my garden, happy with babies and a bright sunshiny future. It should have ended with a song on the wind and a smile on my face and a country hopeful that my recovery meant others, too, could hope to recover from a devastating and deadly illness.

A step on the way to curing mental illness? Even if something that huge were not possible, my recovery would be my happy ending, a personal miracle.

It should have ended with Dad as a success and David recognized for his brilliant, inventive mind. I always pictured Dad standing on a stage filled with lights and flowers, and next to him his dear friend, David. They would be in tuxedos and shiny black shoes, and I would be at the microphone, praising their courage and dedication in the face of brutal criticism and enormous opposition. I would thank them for standing up to these challenges. And I would thank them for taking up the cause of the most misunderstood people in our society: the mentally ill, who cannot stand up for themselves.

In my perfect ending the crowd would cheer. A big trophy would go to Dad and another to David, and they would smile and shuffle in their shiny dress shoes because they aren't comfortable with the adulation. But I would be proud enough for both of them. For the time being, though, I could see that this ending was a long way off. By 2001, it was clear that Canada was not changing the law after all. In fact, the only thing that changed was the Minister of Health. The agreeable Alan Rock was shuffled off to a different position, and a senior cabinet minister, Anne McLellan, took his place. The bureaucrats had found a way around implementing the full fifty-three recommendations that the public had demanded. New rules were coming into play, improving some things, but keeping the old regulations of the Food and Drug Act, which applied restrictions suited to pharmaceutical drugs to natural health products.

In the early days of discovery David had known our only hope of survival under Canadian law would come from science. If our claims could be proven, how could the product be illegal? "No one is going to take the word of a pig-feed guy and an engineer," David said. "I know my place." He always laughed when he said that.

They had seen so much, and yet could prove so little. The changes in Joe and me had now been experienced by people living in the small towns of southern Alberta. The treatment had trickled by word of mouth all across Canada and into the United States; it had crept in narrow streams across England, Norway, New Zealand, and China. As more people came on board, willing to document their symptoms, renowned neurologist Dr. Bryan Kolb saw Dad and David's data.

The data was simply a handful of self-rating forms, multiple-choice questionnaires filled out by the sick person as he or she began switching from drugs to the supplement. But Dr. Kolb took the time to interview me, and he asked to see my medical records for proof that I had been as ill as I claimed. Then he suggested that Dad and David talk to a University of Calgary psychologist named Dr. Bonnie Kaplan, a researcher in the field of behavioural science. She scoffed at first and asked Dr. Kolb not to send them to her.

"Guys, I'm sorry," she said. "I've dealt with all the quacks I can handle in my career. I'm just not interested."

Still, she offered to help Dr. Kolb with some forms for data collection, which Dad and David then proceeded to use with a small group of children. A few months later Dr. Kolb analyzed the data and faxed the results to Dr. Kaplan. She was startled by them and curious, finally, to know more. She phoned Dr. Kolb and said she would like to meet with these men now.

Dad, David, and I went to Calgary to meet with her, and I told her my story in detail. She had studied nutrition and behaviour ten years earlier, and now, her curiosity piqued, she was considering doing research on the supplement. First, however, she followed the case of one child, one who was young enough not to understand the placebo effect or the benefits of faking an illness. As she saw his moods settle and as his violence subdued, she decided to come on board.

Dr. Kaplan put together a preliminary study using the supplements Dad and David had prepared, both the pills and the liquid. They were certain of the combination now because over the first couple of years we had tried several variations: reducing the pills, trying new ones, increasing the liquid. When the supplements got out of balance, I did, too. But it still wasn't clear which of the ninety-two ingredients were actually the active ingredients.

Dr. Kaplan decided to study the entire combination as if it were one ingredient. Never mind which of the minerals and vitamins were working; she reasoned that it was better to study the whole formulation to see if it was working at all and worry about the breakdown later.

She had twelve children in this first trial and documented the results as they went along. When Dr. Kaplan received her second shipment of the supplements, the liquid was different. New and improved, better taste, lighter colour. The results weren't bad, but they weren't good. They appeared to be random.

And with the same liquid in my supplement, I crashed. Dana panicked.

"Hi, Dad. It's Dana . . . Yeah, glad I caught you. Listen, Autumn's sick again. Yeah, of course she's taking the stuff . . . No. Nothing else has changed." He's worried, running his hand over his head and rocking on his feet. "The batch number? Okay, let me get the bottle." I watch him from my pacing, tapping, flapping spot in the living room. He fumbles with the bottles on top of the fridge. He reads the batch number off the bottle to Dad and clutches it by the neck as he paces back to keep an eye on me. "Yeah, it's the light-coloured one. She's been on this stuff for, I don't know, a couple weeks, maybe three." There is a long pause while Dana nods and nods. Then he shakes his head and says goodbye.

"Take more, Autumn. Just take more. Dad says the formula might have changed with the so-called improvements. Lots of people are having trouble. You need to double up."

I drank two bottles, then three, and got up to six bottles a month before Dr. Kaplan and David and Dad figured out what had gone wrong. The small company that produced the liquid had been overwhelmed by the sudden number of orders for the product. They mined the minerals from plant material sealed in the earth, packed full of digestible minerals in dense quantities. The demand was great and the flavour was not, so they found new mines and blended the product.

Dr. Kaplan asked an outside lab to analyze the contents of the bottles, and the results showed differences between batches. The original bottles, dark and bitter, contained minerals in tiny amounts that were not found in the newer tastier product. Dad called the producers and begged them to go back to the original formula.

"Autumn, you won't believe what the president of the company said to me."

"What?"

"The guy says, 'You have no right to conduct research using our product.' So I tell him it's for my kids, and that Dr. Kaplan is interested in proving our findings—right or wrong. But he says to stop using it because it doesn't work to heal bipolar, and he doesn't want to be taken out by the FDA for making a therapeutic claim on a natural product."

Because of this problem, Dr. Kaplan's first trial was a disappointment, and she couldn't set up new research either. She had to wait for Dad and David to come up with a better, stable solution. Dad and David went to work, sifting through stacks of research dating back to the 1930s, absorbing reams of studies, publications from the U.S. Department of Agriculture, and largely depending, once again, on David's pig-feed formulating experience to determine proper ratios between the elements.

David had once made a career out of keeping pigs in top condition. It was good business for pork producers to give the animals supplements. Ironically, financial interest in the industry had taken animal nutrition know-how far beyond human nutrition. After all, no one in the human health industry really benefited when humans worked in top condition. In the human realm, big money is made on sickness, not health.

David took his enthusiasm and focused it on us, giving up the pigs for Joe and me and fifty or so formerly ill neighbours and friends. We happily became David's guinea pigs, trying new combinations and new liquids, and eventually new pills and then new capsules. A lot of new capsules. I was told to take thirty-two capsules a day. Gross.

"Hello, Mr. Hardy?"

"Hello, yes."

"Um, hi. It's Autumn calling. Do you have a minute? I just need to ask you a few questions."

"Sure." I hear him shuffle and settle on the other end of the line.

"How come, when it was liquid, we only needed a couple ounces and a few tablets, and now that it's your stuff, we have to eat thirty-two capsules a day? I can't swallow that many. It's disgusting."

"Autumn, if all we wanted to do was feed you the minerals and vitamins, we could get them into two capsules, but you wouldn't be able to digest them. The capsules would have little or no benefit, like most of the supplements on the market. The reason the first liquid batches worked so well was that they contained minerals from plant sources, naturally chelated, or chemically bonded, in the soil with organic acids and taken up by the ancient plants. But the balance, the ratio of mineral to mineral, was all over the place, and the source was totally unreliable. We had to find a way to get a stable, predictable product and still maintain the digestibility, the bio-availability. So we used an organic chelation process, but it made the product very, very bulky, as you know. It turned two capsules' worth of minerals and vitamins—essential co-factors— into thirty-two capsules."

Forty minutes of explanation was enough for me. I swallowed hard thirty-two times a day and did my best to be consistent. And my health improved beyond the best I had ever been on the liquid combination. Other people were obedient swallowers, too. But many just couldn't do it and had to walk away, going back to their medications. The day that Dad and David released their newest fifteen-capsule-a-day product, I swear I heard a cheer go up across Canada. At least there was a cheer in my home.

In 2001, with a stable, reliable product which Dad and David called EMPowerplus, and a raft of success stories from the local guinea pigs, Dr. Kaplan was able to begin more research, this time with adult subjects. The results were astounding. Eighty percent of the patients who tried the supplement showed a significant reduction in symptoms. And half of them were off their drugs within the first six weeks. This was better than any drug trial she had seen. And she suspected that the supplement might do its work even better and faster if there were no psychotropic drugs involved. The symptoms of withdrawal, addiction, and discontinuation syndrome might be mimicking the illness and skewing the data.

Dr. Kaplan obtained funding from the Alberta government to do a placebo-controlled test. The placebo, a pill with no active ingredients, would go to a control group. The test would serve to prove that subjects like me and Joe and many others weren't just so hopeful about Truehope that we stopped our lunacy by willpower alone. She filed the papers describing a study on the effect of a vitamin and mineral combination and gathered her colleagues, a group of psychiatrists. She developed her protocol and submitted it for peer review, for ethics committee approval. It passed. She found willing patients, and good things were happening everywhere. Dad called to give me an update.

"Hey, kiddo, how's that pregnancy going?"

"Dad, you're back!" I shuffle the phone between my neck and shoulder and set toddling Samantha down on the carpet to play with her blocks. "How was your trip? Was it good?"

"Oh, you bet it was. Are you healthy?"

"Yeah, I'm fine. I'm taking it easy, y'know, eating, staying off my feet. Threatening an early delivery, but that's just me. I'm always in a hurry to get to the finish line. You know that."

"Good, good." He's distant. He's got something to say.

"Okay. Enough stalling. Tell me everything."

"Okay . . . Aww, I wish you could have been there, kiddo, it was fantastic. We flew out to Boston and did a presentation for a boardroom full of doctors. Not just doctors—specialists, the big guys from Harvard."

"Wow! Who spoke?"

"Oh, Bonnie ran the thing. I told the family story, about you and Joe, about Debbie. Then David talked about the data we've been collecting from participants and about the early stuff, the deficiency theory, the development of the supplement. Bonnie presented all her work, the preliminary research. It was powerful!"

"Did they like it? Did they want to help?"

"They were intrigued. Really. Fascinated. I think they saw what we have here. Dr. Charles Popper, the specialist in psychopharm, even took a bottle from David. Said he'd look into Bonnie's work. Said he'd be in touch." I can imagine his excited grin over the phone, his clenched fist. *Yes!*

"Wow! Dad, that's super! You've got the big guns on your side now!"

"It's a blessing. The Lord's with us on this one, Autumn."

"Oh, for sure, Dad. They'll make good on my claim of sanity." I want that validation so badly. Proof that I was once as sick as I was and that I am now as well as I claim to be. Proof that it's possible. I'm tired of being brushed off as an anecdotal testimonial. I want proof.

And Dr. Kaplan came close. That year, with Dr. Popper's help, she published her preliminary findings in the *Journal of Clinical Psychiatry* and invited other university professors to replicate her results. The journal was sent out and she got her first response from the Canadian government.

Health Canada shut her down.

TPD Health Canada, the drug regulation division, determined that she could not study a vitamin and mineral supplement for use on bipolar disorder. By virtue of their policy, based on the unchanged law, the very law that the government had promised to change back when we were fighting over making foods into drugs, all treatments for Schedule A diseases like bipolar, depression, asthma, impotence, and incurable diseases like multiple sclerosis and Parkinson's could, by law, be treated only with drugs. So if EMPowerplus was being used by bipolars and making them well, it was indeed a drug under the law and not a supplement.

Thus Dr. Kaplan's Alberta government–funded research was shut down by unelected bureaucrats in Ottawa, and Dad and David were told to stop selling the supplement, to stop providing it to anyone with mental illness. Right now.

Now that EMPowerplus was classified as a drug, they would need to come up with millions of dollars and pull the product off the market for up to ten years before they would receive a notice of compliance for continued research or a drug identification number in order to sell the new drug in Canada. And even if they did everything asked of them, there was no guarantee that they would be given the approval that was needed to sell a drug in Canada. That would be left up to the discretion of a regulatory body responsible for approving the sale of pharmaceuticals.

Truehope's only hope for validation, the study, had shut down. Minerals and vitamins were only for healthy people, drugs for sick people. Those were the rules. And we would have to live or die by the rules. All of us were to resume standard drug therapy. Therapy that Health Canada said was proven safe and effective.

Our own government had become our enemy.

41

Dad and David had over three thousand Canadians on the supplement, and all had been enjoying the stable product just long enough to feel safe and secure in their new lives. I felt safe. I felt confident. And Dana did, too, confident enough to leave his career as an engineering technologist and move the family south to be closer to my dad and my siblings. He was going to help establish a charity for the mentally ill and a good support system for EMPowerplus users. He worked hard to help my dad and to keep me blissfully out of the loop.

I was wrapped up in a busy normal life and was happy to step back from Truehope. James turned ten, Samantha turned three, and baby Melanie started walking. Then, when I found I was pregnant again, my life was absorbed in mothering and nurturing and nothing else. It was someone else's turn to talk, someone else's turn to be worried. I didn't know then that I ought to be worried.

After all I had been through, I never expected that someone might begrudge me my wellness or think that I was not deserving of my happiness. I thought that being well, being the mother of four kids and a productive member of my community, made my life worth saving. I thought I was way beyond being a disposable statistic, but I wasn't.

My story of recovery was all too easily dismissed as a marketing ploy, and no one seemed to care when Dad said shutting down his business would kill his son and daughter. I caught on to how bad the situation was when friends began calling, asking to borrow supplements because their orders had been turned back at the border. And Dana had to leave his work with the charity and take on a more urgent assignment.

Over the telephone Dad gave directions to Dana like a general marshalling his troops. "I want you on this 24/7. We need letters from participants. Gather up all the ones you already have, and send an e-mail asking for more. If those suckers are shutting this thing down, they'd better know who they are hurting. Don't stop, Dana, don't stop until you have five hundred. Five hundred letters."

"Got it. I'm on it." Dana hung up and went to work. He wrote his letter, and I wrote mine. His parents wrote, begging for mercy for their son and for me: "Please don't make them go back to that."

When they could get no co-operation from the agents and enforcers, Dad and David decided to go above Health Canada and seek a ministerial exemption. They were confident that Anne McLellan, the new Minister of Health, would put a stop to the interference with shipments of EMPowerplus if she knew lives were truly at stake.

Dad wanted a package for her that could not be ignored. He also planned to copy the letters and send them to all the Health Canada agents that were involved in the demand that Truehope be shut down. If they knew how many people were using the supplement, and why, he believed they'd have to concede. Letters poured into Dana's fax machine and e-mail.

When Dad and David went to Ottawa, they were armed with reams of letters and ready to seek an audience with anyone who would listen. But Anne McLellan wouldn't meet them, and ultimately she was the only one who could make a difference.

Soon Dad received another letter, warning him to stop all assistance to the mentally ill and to stop promoting the use of the supplement in Canada. By continuing his mental health support program, he was acting in defiance of Health Canada policy. He reacted angrily, venting his frustration over the phone in every direction he could think of.

When Sandra Jarvis, an agent for Health Canada, started her investigation of Truehope, she posed on the phone as a depressed woman, and the Truehope staffers wanted to help her. So she got what she was looking for.

Yes, it was true, the Truehope support system was encouraging people to use the supplement as a possible solution for depression and bipolar affective disorder.

Yes, they had stories of thousands of Canadians who were dependent on the supplement to maintain mental health.

So, she answered Dad's defiance with a silent show of strength that was easy for her and fellow compliance officer Miles Brosseau. Since the product was produced in the United States, they had the power, under the authority of the Minister of Health, Anne McLellan, to turn back the shipments at the border.

Then they took their investigation a step further and seized a massive shipment. They opened every bottle, breaking the seals and rendering a fortune's worth of the supplement unusable. As shipments stopped coming and supplies dwindled, a panic rose in Canada.

Dad and David redoubled their efforts to come to some agreement with Health Canada, but doors were shut along with the borders, and the word from above was clear. These boys were stepping on sacred policy and that was not to be tolerated. Meanwhile, two suicides were reported. The families blamed the government embargo on the supplement for the loss of their children.

The bureaucrats couldn't have imagined it would be so tough to shut down a tiny rural Alberta company. And those agents were in no way prepared for Dad's hot fury and the verbal lashing they took when he got them on the telephone. It must have been shocking to them that Dad took the shut-down orders so personally. He called the agents by their first names plus a few choice alternatives, and refused to buy it when they tried to duck behind the wall of duty and policy. It's just business, they might have thought. The guy has a good idea, he wants special treatment, he can't get it. He'll have to go through the proper channels, and that takes time. And who cares—it's just vitamins and minerals. It's not as if people can't go to the store and get a different brand.

The government bureaucrats didn't see the Tony and David train coming; they didn't hear the warning bells at the crossing. They should have stepped off the track. Only men with a personal stake could fight the fight the way Dad and David did, and God made sure they were ready, both of them, because by the time the first order to shut down Truehope came, David had two of his thirteen kids diagnosed and fully dependent on the supplement for their normal happy lives.

The day Joanna Goral made the first phone call to tell Dad to shut down his operation, she couldn't have known that it was the equivalent of waging war on the man's family. This was not business, this was survival; not money, but a mission.

Miles Brosseau sent a cease-and-desist order. Dad called me and everyone else to vent.

"I'm not sitting here another minute. I'm not taking this sitting here in Alberta. They want to do this? They're gonna have to say it to my face. Shut down, cease, desist? No bloody way."

He packed a bag and picked up David and they drove twelve hours through the Rocky Mountains to get to Miles and his boss, Dennis Shelley. During the hours on the road David talked Dad into behaving in a courteous manner. So when they got into the meeting, he tried.

C'mon. Let's be reasonable, guys.

Nope. No deal.

Fruitless reasoning brought on frothing anger, and Dennis warned he would take all necessary action to force Dad to shut Truehope down. Dad stood up and yelled in their faces. "We aren't backing down. You aren't shutting us down. You hear me? So, what's next? Should we turn ourselves in to the RCMP on the way out of town?"

It hadn't come to that yet.

All the way home Dad steamed, gripping the steering wheel with one white-knuckled hand, shaking his head, exploding into angry words at regular intervals. Meanwhile, David was composing a seven-page letter, transforming Dad's explosions and spews into a civil but firm warning. They would warn Health Canada of the consequences of shutting down Truehope.

When Dad got home, he stayed up all night with my brothers, faxing that seven-page letter to eight hundred Health Canada offices across the country demanding an answer. Are you prepared to violate human rights to life and liberty and security over this policy? Who exactly are you protecting?

When Dennis Shelley took a leave of absence, Rod Neske took over Shelley's spot and sent a cease-and-desist order to Truehope. In response,

Dad grabbed the phone and threatened a lawsuit, personal financial ruin and criminal and civil accountability.

The government took the next step and blocked shipments of EMPowerplus from the manufacturer in the United States. Customs agents seized supplement bottles at the border. Dad was finished. Or so the bureaucrats thought.

Nope. He called in the press and announced his intention to sue the Attorney General of Canada and the Minister of Health.

It wasn't that they were threatening his business; he didn't care about that. They were threatening his children. Sending me to a psych ward was as good as handing me a vacuum hose and a van. Taking the supplement away from Joe was as good as turning Dad's home into a hell. Denying his children and grandchildren access to his miracle was like killing the love of his life, Debbie, all over again.

42

My brother Daniel, famous for his pranks and practical jokes, was given the task. His mission? To find phone numbers. If the government officials at Health Canada didn't want to meet, then he'd find them in their homes and offices. Anne McLellan, the Minister of Health, was top of Dad's list because she had the authority to stop the agents from withholding the supplement. Dad was determined to find a way to get the message to her and all the others, too. And if the policy worshippers weren't going to answer the phone at the office, maybe they'd pick it up at home or at the cabin on the lake. If Dad wasn't sleeping, then none of them would be sleeping.

Phone calls rang out from the homes of supplement users to the homes and offices and weekend cabins of supplement withholders all across Canada. There were hundreds of Truehope participants, again sending letters, making phone calls, demanding change, begging for mercy; reminding the government that this battle had already been fought and won before Alan Rock was shuffled to another job. But no one in Health Canada or the office of the Minister of Health would listen.

Still, some orders were slipping through the border legally, and others were being smuggled through by desperate people like Dana. He tried not to talk about it. He drove over the border and lied to bring bottles back for me. He didn't tell me much about the battle that was raging. Dana tried hard to spare me the stress and let me get through the pregnancy happily.

But Dad can't help himself. He has to let me know what is going on.

After hearing it, I decide it's time for me to pick up the phone. Surely the situation can't be as bad as Dad says.

"Anne McLellan's office." The woman on the other end of the phone sounds harried.

"My name is Autumn Stringam. I'm calling with a concern about the availability of a vitamin and mineral supplement here in Canada. Apparently it is being called an illegal drug."

"Ma'am, are you calling about Truehope?"

"Yes . . ."

"A mental health crisis line has been set up to address your needs."

"But—" The phone clicks in my ear, and I'm left murmuring to myself, I'm not in a mental health crisis.

At least she didn't hang up. The phone rings twice. A different voice answers.

"This is Chantelle. How can I help you?"

"Hi, Chantelle. I just called the Minister of Health because my vitamins are being kept out of Canada and called an illegal drug." I'm very composed, very cool. "They turned me over to you. I don't need counselling, Chantelle. I just want some answers about availability and the warnings about EMPowerplus."

"Yes. This line has been commissioned by the Minister of Health to help people who used to use that drug." She's reading from a script—rote, dry, bureaucratic drivel.

"I still am using it. And it's not a drug. It's a food supplement, vitamins and minerals. I've been using it for seven-and-a-half years."

"Yes, well, it is no longer legal to consume that drug in Canada, so you will not be able to get it into Canada after your supply runs out, ma'am."

"I don't understand. Why are vitamins and minerals suddenly an illegal drug?" I know the answer, but I won't stand for it. This food supplement is not a drug.

But that's just my opinion, according to her. "EMPowerplus is a drug," she insists. "The manufacturers have not provided proof of safety, and Health Canada has identified a risk in consuming it. It will not be permitted to enter Canada until the company provides scientific proof of this drug's safety and efficacy." Chantelle is stiff, fully scripted.

"Um, okay, we are talking about vitamins and minerals—not a drug. What's the risk?"

"The risk?"

"Yes. What risk have they identified? How is it dangerous for me to eat this, this . . . this food?" A long silence ensues. The script did not prepare her for this question. I hear Chantelle typing. And I hear her mumbling.

Finally she comes back, sounding justified. "I have just looked up the warning on the Health Canada Web site. It is a Type Two Risk."

"Type Two. What does that mean?"

"Ma'am, I don't know. They have not given me that information."

"Chantelle?" I hold on to the desk and the phone and set my jaw. I will not be shrill. I will not let Chantelle believe that I am a crazy person. I will not behave like one.

"Yes?"

"You just told me—a pregnant woman who has been healthy for seven-and-a-half years—that the vitamins I've been using to maintain my mental health are now an illegal drug because of a risk so terrible that it warrants their seizure at the border. But you can't tell me what that risk is?"

"I'm sorry, I—"

"I want to know. I have given birth to two healthy daughters while taking this supplement, and I don't believe for a second that the risk exists. Perhaps they ought to be more concerned about the risk of alcohol consumption or overdose of psych meds or Tylenol. People die every day using those things. People don't die eating vitamins and minerals. You know that. Even if there were some mysterious risk, it wouldn't amount to anything, next to the side effects of the crap they had me taking in the hospital."

"Ma'am, can I have your name?"

"Why?" My heart starts pounding.

"I'd like to find some answers and call you back." I have visions of the call-back, paranoid visions. The police will show up at my door to take the certifiable pregnant woman into psych ward custody. I have visions of three doctors nodding and looking over my history. They all sign the bottom of the paper to agree that I must be forced to go back to safe and effective treatments, not like the risky unapproved drug I am taking now.

The male nurse comes and holds me down while they slip the multi-coloured bracelet onto my wrist. Next will come the psychotropic drugs in a needle full of sleep.

I don't want that call-back. I have not been away from those experiences long enough to forget them. I will never forget them.

I won't give my name to Chantelle. I can't. I'm not so brave I'd ever risk going back there. And now my cheeks are hot, and I feel the tears streaming down my face. I can't go back.

"Ma'am?"

"I don't think you can get the answers to my questions, Chantelle. I know this is a crappy job for you. I'm sorry. I know none of this is your fault." *But I can't go back to insanity.*

"Thank you. I'd like to be more help."

"Yes, but you can't be."

Chantelle wishes me luck and hopes I will seek medical attention when I get sick again. *When*, not *if*.

I hang up and drop my head on the desk. I breathe through a contraction. I know it's a fake contraction. This baby is not due for another four months, but today we are both having an internal fit. A wave of helpless rage takes me, and I want to stomp and demand and plead and wail and command attention. The way I used to. But I can't do that. I can't prove Health Canada right.

I don't wail, but I do call Dad, and he puts David on the line as well, and they listen while I dial the helpline and talk it all over with Chantelle again. This time Dad records the whole conversation. He says he'll use it some day, when he gets his day in court. That's all Dad can hope for, a day in court, because right now no one is listening. He is realizing that he is powerless to protect me from this government. It's time to try a new approach.

43

Dad tried to give me my assignment on the phone, but I was not co-operative. I laughed and said no. And then I got angry and said NO. So he invited Dana and me out to dinner and brought a crowd of relatives with him. He knew how to approach an edgy pregnant woman who was threatening another early delivery. In a very public place, among many witnesses, where he was sure I'd be rational.

"You have to get up and go and do something about this."

"Dad. I'm supposed to be on bedrest."

"There are hundreds of people running out of supplement, and two reported dead. You people need to get together and help yourselves."

"Like what, do what?"

"Look, if Gandhi can take down a whole government with salt and a starvation campaign, you can solve this problem."

"That's ridiculous, Dad. I'm not Gandhi." It's just me. Autumn. And I'm pregnant and tired, and I just want to be home with my kids.

I'm a coward, hiding behind my new life. My very busy life and my doctor's order of rest and relaxation. I used to hide behind my madness. Now that I'm normal, I have to hide behind normal things. I have every excuse to stay home.

The waiter comes by to take orders, and I take the time to regroup. I am thinking about ways to refuse his request. Nope, I just can't do it, Dad. I'm no Gandhi. Just say no. He knows he is asking too much.

Waiting for our meal, we try to chat politely with each other, but the air is dense with tension.

"I can't fight this for you any more." Dad blurts it out two minutes after the salads have arrived.

"What?"

The salad tumbles from his fork as he raises it. But even when he gets a bite to his mouth, he doesn't stop talking to chew it. "To the bureaucrats, I'm not the desperate dad any more, Autumn, no matter what the threat is to our family. They'll always see me as an owner, a guy with a business to protect. If you and all the others want this stuff available in Canada, you are going to have to take a stand."

Dad is relentless. "Autumn, I felt it this morning before I called you." He taps his chest with his fingertips. "This one is your problem. You have to go to Ottawa. You get a bunch of women together, and you get there by Tuesday. The House of Commons closes for the summer on Friday, so you have to be there on Tuesday."

He never gives up. If he had given up on me, I wouldn't be here, breaking his heart.

"Dad, but I . . ." All eyes at the table are on Dad now. The chewing has stopped and the forks have dropped. He puts down his glass and leans forward, his hands pressed flat on either side of his plate.

"If you do this, He will bless you, Autumn. You'll be okay. Your baby will be okay. Your family will be okay. I can't fight this one, not for you or any of the others. This one is up to you."

"Okay, Dad. I'll do it."

Five days later I am standing in the wind, the sound of new friends all around me. My heart is throbbing with a fresh dose of pure adrenaline. My cell phone rings.

"What are you doing?" It's Dad.

"I can't talk right now, Dad. The TV cameras from Global just arrived."

"What's going on?" He's talking with an echo, and I know he has me on speaker phone.

"Right now we are nine women on Parliament Hill with red umbrellas."

I hear screaming and cheering, clapping. My Aunt Noelle and Uncle Elward, my brothers Dan and Brad, my dad and David Hardy are all huddled around the speaker.

"Good! I knew it, Autumn. I knew you could do it!"

"They're getting ready to film. I gotta go."

"We're praying for you."

"Thanks, Dad, love ya."

"Love ya, too, bye."

With the arrival of cameras, the Members of Parliament were more than happy to join us. They called to us: Ladies with Red Umbrellas, what are you here for? We would smile and wave, and they would join us to hear our stories and sympathize with our plight. And our red umbrellas had grabbed their attention, too. The night before, we had met with two Members of Parliament and discovered that no one would be able to help us immediately, unless Anne McLellan would intervene on our behalf and give a ministerial exemption. The next morning I woke early and stood in the hotel window, watching the rain fall and feeling completely hopeless. How could we ever get them to notice us when Anne wouldn't meet with us and all of our contacts were tapped out? I had a vision of all of us on Parliament Hill with umbrellas, shivering and huddling and waiting, and then saw the vision another way. I decided to buy red umbrellas and make the problem work in our favour. We called the press and told them to watch for us. We'd be waiting for Anne to notice us.

"Who would you like to see most?" an older MP who noticed our red umbrellas asked me. His cowboy belt told me he was from the West.

"I need to get this problem resolved, so I want to see the people who can change the situation and not just talk about it. I want to see the Minister of Health, Anne McLellan."

"I'll go ask Anne why she won't see you."

The MP came back an hour later. "She said that she doesn't meet with terrorists."

Another Member of Parliament, Dr. James Lunney, did help. He decided to sponsor a press conference for us. But we would have to wing it. No rehearsal, no script. Exactly one half-hour in front of eight national cameras, from the Charles Lynch room, the one with the stage and all of the flags, in the heart of the most powerful building in Canada.

This was our moment, our one chance to prove our sanity, to prove our point, to say it all, to all of Canada, and to be heard.

Half an hour before the press conference we started getting sick with nerves. Asking ourselves and each other questions: What will we say? What can we do? We felt stress and fear, unbelievable fear. So much was at stake.

Desperate to collect ourselves and having nowhere to do it, we stood in a circle on the sidewalk, our umbrellas surrounding us and guarding us from onlookers. And we prayed. Bless our efforts, give us courage, give us strength, open our mouths, and let us speak.

Then we left our umbrellas, passed through security, and stepped into the lights on the stage. We spoke, spontaneously stepping forward, pushed by a strength and composure that we didn't know we had before this moment. And we filled the half-hour exactly. We were no longer fragile, we were no longer cute. When it was my turn, I said we were the new face of mental illness in Canada. We didn't look crazy. We were just moms and wives and women making sense.

The national news took a different view.

We gathered on the hotel bed and watched a forty-second spot about us at the end of the broadcast. They did not show the formal press conference, not even a sound bite. They showed women on edge before speaking. They showed us frowning and scowling at the weather. They showed the prime minister getting into his limo, ignoring us. They showed Sabine fumbling to take her supplement. They showed file photos of infants with horrible birth defects. They said I was pregnant and taking an unapproved drug.

Their message: This was a dangerous choice, and Health Canada had posted a Type Two Risk warning against using EMPowerplus.

From that day on it seems to me that this battle never ends. I live in two worlds, my garden and my battlefield. The two rarely mix or even notice each other. In my garden life I am a mother. I am a wife. In my garden life I am patient and kind and full of compassion. I am soft. I am busy.

In my battlefield life I am the new face of mental illness. No longer ill.

I am bold and determined and sometimes I am angry. In my battlefield life I think about the fight with the Canadian government, my survival, access to the supplement, plans to assist the mentally ill when all the fighting is over.

Then it's early October 2003, and I really don't want to leave my garden life for the exhausting battlefield of Ottawa, but it's a battle I cannot abandon. Red Umbrella Suzanne says that even if she is there alone, she will go to support Dr. Lunney. He has proposed a change in law that will clear the way for me and Joe and every other consumer of natural health products. It won't pass. I'm sure of that. I don't want to go. I'm afraid of failure, and I am tired of fighting. Baby Meagan is barely six weeks old. My garden life is all I want right now. My garden needs me.

Dana won't hear of it. He wants me to go and support Dr. Lunney's bill. Red Umbrella Sheila agrees. She'll come, too. We decide that we'll see this through to the end, no matter what the outcome. We spend two days on Parliament Hill, lobbying and reminding the officials. We share our story once again. We pass out lapel pins to MPs, embossed with shiny red umbrellas, and we ask them to vote for Lunney's bill. Then we fly all night and drive all morning and I get back home. I'm exhausted but happy to be back in my garden world again. Today, however, my garden will meet my battlefield in a clash of images.

I curl up in the living room. I pull my hair up into a high ponytail and lean back against the soft cushions of the worn green couch. I'm warm in pyjama pants and a big sweat shirt. I hear James tromping up the driveway and pushing through the door. I look up to see him as he comes around the corner. My Little Boy Blue has grown. He is tall and dimpled and blond. He is broad and thick, and his feet are bigger than Dana's. He is eleven. And now he can stand flat-footed and look me in the eye.

"Mom!"

"James, I'm so glad to see you." He comes for a kiss and a squeeze and plops down beside me.

"How was the trip?"

"Fine, I'm just glad to be home."

"I missed you. What are you watching?"

"I missed you, too. It's CPAC." The parliamentary channel. "I want to watch the vote on Bill C-420."

"Huh, that's boring."

"We've been fighting for it for years, James. Since you were four."

"Are you winning?"

"Not this time. But we will. Eventually."

James humours me and watches the television. I start to watch, too, until I am distracted by a fairy princess flitting in from the kitchen and twirling on the carpet in her ballet slippers. Samantha, in her favourite purple chiffon dress. She is graceful in her four-year-old body. Her wide blue eyes show her happiness that Mom is home. She is a constant reminder to me that there is life after mental illness.

I remember when I wasn't so sure of that, when I wondered if this normal life was too good to be true. And there were times when I came close to losing it, during my pregnancies. I recall times when I had to remind myself that even normal women struggle sometimes; normal women feel stress. Normal women have hormones, too. As long as I had my supplement, I was normal. And today I and others were losing the battle for protection one more time.

"Are those your pins?" James is still here beside me, and I can barely see the TV for all of the dancing in front of it. Samantha has now been joined by a second fairy princess, white-blonde Melanie, with eyes like Angie's and a body like Sunni's.

"What?" I lean in to see the shining ovals on the lapels of the men and women who are standing to vote Yea. "Oh, my gosh. Those *are* our pins. Red Umbrella pins. Count them, James, count the Yea votes."

Samantha and Melanie dance in front of the television, so we lose count. But I don't care. I've been away, and my girls are the only victory I need to see today. I console myself in their dance. Health Canada can't take that away from me. Baby Meagan coos beside me and draws my attention away from the dance and the TV. I have to smile; this room is full of my children.

James is cheering for the Yea votes and the pins. It seems that there are Yea votes where they weren't expected to be, and pins everywhere.

James is yelling at the TV as if it's a hockey game. The Nay votes are standing to be counted. The girls are oblivious in their fairy-princess dance, laughing and chasing and tripping on their dresses. I hold Meagan against my chest and realize I am squeezing her too hard. Entire rows of Liberals stand to defend the unfair law. They pat each other on the back; they smile when the Opposition yells at them. My daughters flit and flutter in front of the screen trailing lace and ribbon and tulle.

Then I see Anne McLellan. She nods to confirm her vote of Nay. The Opposition roars. And I roar, joining the battle. "Sit down. How can you seem so cold? You are supposed to be helping people, not making vitamins into drugs. Sit down!"

My girls have stopped dancing to watch me. So I check myself. I pass Meagan to James and stop yelling. It's not hockey after all.

The camera pans about the room and settles on the Speaker. He rises to read the results. I reach for the remote to turn the TV off after the tally. I'll explain this failure to James, but I can't bear to see Anne celebrate her victory.

The Speaker speaks: "I declare the motion carried."

What? "What did he say?" *What did he just say?*

The numbers come up on the screen: *Yeas* 124, *Nays* 85.

Gravity has no hold on me. I am in the air. James is on his feet. My floppy pyjama pants wave over my girls' heads as I leap around the room.

"We won! James, James, we won!" I am crying, and James is laughing and crying with me, and the girls are watching and wondering if they should cry with us both. I rush to them to assure them that Mommy is okay.

I spin the girls and kiss James and dance on the carpet and the couch. And then I come to myself. How can it be? How can it be that I am here after all that has happened to me: her garden, the bat, the goat, her life, The Peace Country, Grimshaw, Fort McMurray, hell. And more: her death, her closet, my illness, the drugs, the visions, the demons, Dad's discovery, the dirty laundry, the withdrawal, the recovery, the sorrow, the healing.

"We won. Mom, we won. I can't believe we won!"

My James stands in the middle of the room, tears on his face and his baby sister in his arms. He sees more than just the vote today, too. He understands. He has seen me in the past. The phone rings and cheers echo across Canada. Women take a break from their normal lives, cooking supper and caring for their children, to scream and cry and laugh for joy. Later I sneak off to my room to steal a moment of peace and gratitude. I kneel by my bed. "Thank you," I whisper. "Thank you for letting me live to see this day."

44

It would be pleasant to be able to say that the story ended there. But no. The only thing that ended was the majority Liberal government's reign in Canada. The Liberals won a minority government and Anne McLellan became the Deputy Prime Minister and the Minister of Public Safety. The Honourable Pierre Pettigrew took her place as Minister of Health. Within weeks Pettigrew had met with Dr. Lunney and arranged a deal. Finally, a ministerial exemption was granted and access to the supplement was established legally once again. Dana was relieved that he would not have to act as a smuggler for my personal stash of vitamins and minerals any more.

Then there was another election, and Canadians voted Anne McLellan right out of her seat in the House. But they also got rid of all the unfinished business, including Dr. Lunney's bill and the committee that was to review the proposed change in the law.

In January 2004 new regulations for natural health products came into play. Truehope applied for a regulation number called an NPN, or Natural Product Number. And the product was no longer under the regulatory authority of TPD Health Canada. Dr. Kaplan was allowed to start her research again, and everything was clear sailing for one year.

One year. That's how long it took the government to sift through the boxes of seized papers and junk and computer files to come up with criminal charges against Dad and David. And it would take another two years still before a court date was set.

Eventually, my ever-feisty father came to see this as an opportunity. "If they go through with these charges, then I will get my day in court. I will get to stand up, on public record, and tell my story, the whole thing. All the parts they have never heard and refuse to listen to. I'm gonna have my day in court!"

He and David ran up travel and lawyer bills that would have been enough to provide free supplement to hundreds of sick people. To Dad, that seemed like a terrible waste. When Health Canada agents called, just days before the trial, to say that they were dropping all the charges, Dad went a little nuts.

"So, I called Dennis Shelley and I says, Hey, are you telling me that you sent the RCMP in, seized all our stuff, paid a bunch of public servants to sift through it for years, and that's all you can come up with? Nothing? You are a waste of taxpayers' resources, and you make me sick. You aren't worth your pay, and let me tell you, when I am done cleaning up with your buddies, I'm going to come after you for damages, personally. This has amounted to nothing more than harassment for years, and you will pay for this. *You* will. Not your department."

"You *said* that?" I'm holding the phone and staring at a wall.

"Yeah."

"Like on an answering machine?" *Please say no!*

"No, to Dennis right over the phone."

"And?"

"Well, about half an hour later Shawn Buckley, Truehope's lawyer, calls me, spitting mad, and he tells me to stay off the phone because now they *aren't* going to drop all of the charges. They figure they can get me on selling without a Drug Identification Number."

"So, we *are* going to court?"

"Yeah, and David is not happy about it. He chewed a strip off me over this and what it's going to cost the company. He says I should have let them drop the charges."

"Yes, well, you should have, Dad. None of us want to get dragged through that. For what? What's the worst they can do over a DIN charge?"

"I don't know, maybe five hundred bucks."

"You are going to pay maybe half a million to save yourself five hundred?"

"Okay, you don't get it either. They actually think I'm just an idiot out here trying to protect a measly little vitamin company. I want the whole thing exposed, all of it, the discovery, the research, the shut-downs, the raid. I want you to tell your story—and the other Red Umbrella women, too, telling what they've been put through. These brainless bureaucrats need it on record what they have done, what their sacred policy has done. People have died, Autumn."

"But Dad, you were selling without a DIN, so what kind of defence can you possibly have?"

"Necessity. We acted of necessity. Debbie's death and your getting so sick, and Joe, and the discovery—all necessary. And my fighting like an idiot with these closed-minded people for the last ten years—it's all been necessary for change."

He's changing my mind.

"This battle is what I'm here for. It's my job to change the law, to end this psychiatric hell. They can't stop us. They never should have tried to. It's all necessary. The judge will see that. It's not about a stinking DIN. It's about telling the truth and getting everything on public record. I need your support." I hear his voice crack, and my eyes fill with tears.

Dad's awkward in his anger, but he's right. I know that David will get over his anger with Dad, and he'll sit next to him and fight beside him. We all will. He's right, and he's going to court for the right reasons.

I wipe my tears. "You've got it, Dad. I'll give this battle everything I've got."

"Thanks. Now here's what I need you to do . . ."

45

The oak double doors of the Calgary courtroom are heavy as I push them open to leave. Today Dad is on trial, next to his friend David, and everyone is there for him. I am, too, but I've just been told I can't be with him, can't hear or see the proceedings. Before the lawyer's opening arguments, the judge asked me to leave so that my testimony would not be influenced by others' perspectives. I must wait for my turn to testify, and my turn will not come for days.

I stand up, nod to Dad, *Good luck*, then Dana catches my hand and gives it a squeeze. Dana, like every other person in the packed courtroom, is heavily invested in the outcome of this trial. Years ago he gave up his career in engineering to join Dad and David's efforts to help the mentally ill. Now we work together: He runs the charity, and I help train the staff. We are happy as a team, raising our family. And we both want to be able to go home and tell the children that Grandpa is not a criminal after all.

I pass the benches stuffed with faces, all sympathetic to my ejection from the room. They know I want to be here so badly. But I know they'll support Dad for me; they'll tell me what they saw and heard.

As it turns out, I'll hear plenty of opinions in the days to come, and then I'll have to read eighteen hundred pages of written transcript to form my own. But I'm getting ahead of myself.

I press through the double doors. The sound of my high heels on the stone floor fills the empty atrium lobby, bouncing from the wall to the floor-to-ceiling windows and elevator shafts on my right, echoing over the waist-high glass walls on my left. A few plants are the only organic thing that might soften the space, but they don't absorb the echoes from the floor, and their breath is hardly enough to fill this space that has been sucked free of oxygen by defensive panic. This place reminds me of a hospital I once lived in.

I turn back to the doors and squint through the peephole: it's a view rounded and magnified to expose the broad courtroom through a quarter-inch of glass. There he is, my father, sitting facing the judge, his wife Barb on one side of him and David on the other. Dad's lawyer, the black-haired, slim Shawn Buckley, is standing, one hand in his suit pocket, the other holding the podium from which he will give his first address. The judge is sitting high on his platform. He's far from the door, and his expressions are blurred by distance.

I can't hear a word, and this view cannot satisfy any of my wants, so I turn away, pacing and clicking on the stone floor. Now what? I toss my bag and my red umbrella onto the seat closest to the door. I sink into the institutional leather just as another woman comes out of the courtroom. I look up and my heart sinks.

I recognize her. Dad pointed her out to me this morning. Sandra Marie Jarvis. At first I thought he was joking. Sandra is an average-looking person in practical shoes. Not a monster; not even mean looking. How did she manage to become someone who could strike fear into my heart? How did she manage to become an enemy to Dad?

I peer sideways to see Sandra sitting only a couple of seats over, gripping her notebook with both hands. She flips a page, and I see that it is brimming, top to bottom, with dates and numbers and comments. She looks at me, and I turn the other way and shake my head and I can't believe the fight has gone this far. I can't believe that we are here at all.

But it was Sandra's job to enforce policy, to cut off access to Dad's supplement at the border. If Truehope didn't shut down when commanded, then she'd do it by force. She was just doing her job. That's all any of them were doing.

It doesn't matter who you are or what you stand for. Success, fame, discovery, or change. Detractors have to have work, too. And, of course, Truehope found detractors. The name alone, Truehope, was enough to raise ire. Did that mean other options for treating bipolar were—Falsehope? And who did Dad and David think they were? They were largely uneducated in all things concerning mental health. David knew pig feed. Dad knew loss. The only experience they'd had in mental illness was bad experience. The only experience Dad had in medicine was that medicines didn't always work and never worked for long.

Had they been educated in state-of-the-art modern medicine, however, they never would have been humble enough to look in a pigpen for an answer. Such a modest beginning for such a miraculous discovery. Worthy of detractors and doubters. Worthy of an over-exuberant application and enforcement of policy. Worthy of persecution and prosecution, because no one wants change and the earth should always be flat for the mentally ill.

These are confrontational thoughts and I'm not really that way, even when faced with one who has held my life in her hands and seemed to disregard it. In the mall or on the street I would never give this woman a second glance, and I am not afraid of the outcome of this trial. After all, since Health Canada dropped five of the six charges, we are accused only of selling a drug without a drug identification number, a DIN, and at the worst, in this case the punishment might amount to a five hundred dollar fine. This fight is not about my safety or access to the supplement any more, because the ministerial exemption still stands. Sandra Jarvis lost her authority over my life long ago. Now we are fighting about principle, and that's more important.

The bailiff comes to the door and calls her. "Ms. Jarvis?" She pushes up from her chair and straightens her waistband and clicks past me. I watch her disappear through the courtroom doors and sigh with relief. I shift in my seat and flip through my notebook. I want to write, but I can't. Not here. Not in this frame of mind.

I pick up my umbrella and finger the soft red fabric. That first day on Parliament Hill brought me out, made me bold, gave me courage and hope. I can see now that my dad sent me on a mission that did more for my character than any experience I could have dreamed up on my own. I am driven by my friendships with the other Red Umbrellas to do more, make the most of my experience and bless others' lives with what I have learned. I ought to thank Sandra for that. There's always a silver lining if you look hard enough. Right?

The courtroom doors open frequently as friends come out to walk or pace or sit next to me in a soft chair and give me a summary of the testimony inside.

Sandra Jarvis' testimony is truthful and long and proves that Dad and David have, in fact, been selling the supplement. That the product was produced in the United States and ordered by individuals through Truehope and that the label does not have a drug identification number on it. Why? Because Truehope has been selling the supplement without a DIN. It takes a long time to come around to what everyone already knows.

Just when I think my head will burst with boredom, Dana comes out of the courtroom. He walks with me to the cafeteria and gives me the best report he can come up with.

"So, the prosecution didn't give us anything we didn't know, but the cross-examination brought out a little nugget for you." He grabs a tray and we load our sandwiches on it.

"What? What's the nugget?"

"Ohh, it's gonna make you mad. Remember that Type Two Risk on the Health Canada Web site?" He passes a bill to the cashier.

"Yeah. The one the call line girl told me about. The reason they had to shut down the borders."

"Right. Type Two means 'a remote risk of harm.' Less harmful than baby aspirin. Remote as in not very likely to hurt anyone."

"But Global News cited that warning next to pictures of deformed babies when they said I was pregnant and using an unapproved drug. That's all a Type Two Risk means?"

"Dirty agenda, eh?"

"Makes you wonder, doesn't it?"

As a group we eat lunch in a student cafeteria at the college across the street from the courthouse. When we've finished, we spend the rest of the hour standing in the wind outside the courthouse in a cluster of bright red umbrellas. This time I'm not scared, and I don't need a plan.

This is just about making a show of support for Dad and for David. When we are all thoroughly chilled, we go back inside. Everyone else files back into the courtroom, and I resume my place in the squishy comfortable chair. I need to rethink my involvement. Since sitting here isn't doing anyone a bit of good, I'll go home tonight and take care of the kids. Dana agrees and promises to keep me updated on the phone.

Next up on the stand was the infamous Miles Brosseau, infamous to me only because Dad made him so at Truehope meetings and even family gatherings. He's another Sandra, responsible for shutting down the western borders, unresponsive to pleas for help, even pleas for mercy when Dad drove all night to beg him for understanding on behalf of the Truehope participants in Canada. And Miles travelled to see Dad, too, on a day when Truehope wasn't expecting company.

I'd heard Miles' name so often—associated with such fear and anger— that I might have expected Osama Bin Laden to enter the courtroom. Dana said he had a lumbering walk and looked burdened for time, as if giving testimony was the very last thing he wanted to be doing. He was also a slow speaker. But Dana quickly became Miles' new number one fan.

"It was hilarious." Dana is telling me the details over the phone, and he can hardly contain his laughter. "He cleared the courtroom, it was so boring. He must have been well coached, y'know—like, take your time answering questions, don't be pressured. Don't answer until you've thought it through. Don't give more information on cross-examination than you have to . . . But I'm telling ya, this guy took caution to a whole new level!"

"Like what?" I am wishing I could have been there. Oh, it's a writer's dream come true to have hours to examine such an odd character.

"Like, Buckley asks, 'So if you were sent a document showing that people were dying because of what Health Canada was doing, you would just ignore that information because it's not a policy or a directive?' and Brosseau sits there. No part of his body moves. He just sits there in silence, staring just past Buckley's head—like, forever. Just when you think he's had a seizure or something must be terribly wrong, he grunts a one-word answer."

"What was his answer?"

"He said 'Yes.' Your dad is furious about it. This guy was responsible for shutting off the product at several border crossings, and even knew about the suicides that the CMHA reported, and didn't change what he was doing. He made like he didn't have any responsibility or authority to think for himself."

I feel sick. "Bureaucracy."

I manage to get some sleep, followed by a restful morning, and then the phone rings once more.

It's Shawn Buckley on the line. "They wrapped up prosecution today, and I need you to come back up to Calgary. Your dad is going on first, but I need you to be here. Dress for court, okay? With all of these witnesses lined up, I never know how long the proceedings will take, and I need you as a standby in case I can fit you in."

I know this guy is stressed, working all day, preparing witnesses and newly discovered evidence all night, and when I was taking my EMPowerplus the other day, he asked for some.

"I'll be there."

I pack up the suitcases, bathe three girls, secure the house, pull James from school, and we all drive to Calgary. As I'm driving, Dana calls to tell me about a new word.

"Undiscoverable." He laughs.

"What does that mean?"

"The women on the call line, the counsellors hired to tell you that you couldn't get the supplement any more? They had to keep notes, a record of every call with names and phone numbers: what the complaint was, what the conversation was about. Shawn asked Health Canada to produce the papers as evidence in the trial, and dad's prosecutor, Mr. Brown, has just announced that they are undiscoverable." Dana stops, breathes, and then hisses, "Health Canada agents were hurting people and they want to hide it."

"You have to be kidding. Now what?"

"The judge ordered them to find the call records and produce them for the trial. Now."

"I doubt they will. They won't produce them if they think the records will hurt their case."

"They have to, Autumn . . . When are you getting here?"

"I'm still two hours away."

"Okay. Love Only."

Dana meets me and the kids in the hotel parking lot, hands me the room key, and gets in the driver's seat. The first thing he tells me is that the undiscoverable records have been found, within two hours of the judge's demand that they be produced.

"We'll have them tonight, and Shawn wants us to help sort them, find the highlights."

"That's good stuff, eh?"

"Oh, babe, those calls, if the call line employees took notes properly, those hundreds of calls could make it look really bad for Health Canada. If hundreds of people were saying what you were feeling, it's gotta look pretty bad that the government kept holding up the supplement at the border. And that evidence works for your dad and David. How could they shut down Truehope when people were crying and saying they would die without the supplement? Policy is not a licence to kill."

I kiss him goodbye and watch him drive off with the girls. James and I head up to the room and settle for the night. James will stay and watch court proceedings for the next few days. Dana will drive all night to drop the girls off in Sherwood Park at his parents' house, then return to hear Dad testify the next morning. He does his part, arrives safely, and slides into bed next to me to catch four hours of sleep before the alarm wakes us.

Days go by, and I am still in my place in the courthouse lobby, waiting for my turn, all dressed up with nowhere to go. I have missed Dad's testimony, his chance to tell his side, full of emotion; and the testimony of fellow Red Umbrella Debra O., who stood up for her son and his right to be well. Her testimony was educated, clinical, and motherly all at once. She was tear-stained as she left the courtroom. And I missed an incredible day of Dr. Kaplan explaining her independent university research and defending the necessity of studying the Truehope program. And now I am going to miss Mr. Ron LaJeunesse.

Mr. LaJeunesse. I know him by reputation, and I love what he stands for. He is committed to protecting the rights of the mentally ill, allowing dignity and personal choice in treatment. He developed Alberta's mental health programs and wrote a book promoting the death of stigma. He recently retired from being the head of the Alberta chapter of the Canadian Mental Health Association, but not before he went to bat for a lot of Truehope participants who were running out of the supplement. Ron fought within the system while Dad was fighting in the trenches. I remember some dirty fighting in the trenches. The worst was a raid on Truehope by Sandra Jarvis and Miles Brosseau, almost two years ago.

Sandra and Miles were both there in Raymond, Alberta, the morning the RCMP and Health Canada compliance officers raided the Truehope office. The police came in, fully armed, demanding that all the staff take off their headsets and put their hands on the desks.

I imagine the scene like a cartoon version of *Magnum PI*. The officer is swaggering and cool, and desperate to be obeyed.

Hang up and step away from your telephones. Now.

The person on the other end of the line is already spending the day terrified and paranoid. Imagine the fear of those callers who hear the invasion over the phone.

Put your hands on the desk. You, petite forty-something with the warm fuzzy sticker on your monitor and the picture of your kids on your desk, Stop helping people immediately and go directly to the lunch room. Move it.

Well, maybe not, but they did herd the employees into the lunch room.

Sandra and Miles and all the other agents began demanding names and company positions. They thought they were dealing with staff hired to fill orders. They didn't know that every person there used the product and had felt the very personal threat when they were told too bad, EMPowerplus was not available any more. Please seek medical attention when you get sick again.

This staff had spent months comforting panicked participants, begging people not to follow through on threats of suicide—If I have to go back to drugs, I'll just kill myself.

The staff had felt hopeless coming to work under the Truehope sign day after day, unable to help themselves or their program participants because policy was taking precedence.

This was not business for the participants and it wasn't business for the staff. EMPowerplus was not just another vitamin bottle. It was a matter of life or death. So when the staff knew the agents' names, they cursed them and refused to give passwords, keys, and information. Sandra and Miles must have been shocked.

And when the agents opened the giant industrial warehouse doors, expecting to find a massive EMPowerplus dissemination empire, they must have been disappointed. The warehouse was not a gold mine of criminal activity. It was a personal storage shack for the staff, filled with picnic tables and a couple of donated barbecues, supplies for staff birthday celebrations, a washing machine and clothes dryer, an old couch and some boxes loaded with pots and pans. And, way at the back, David Hardy's family camper.

When the agents hauled out boxes of financial papers, notebooks, and staff training manuals, and found the Photoshopped portrait that my brother Dan distributed of Anne McLellan, complete with horns and a goatee, they knew they must be right about the Truehopers.

The raid lasted only a day, but it was a great Health Canada success when the press reported that Truehope had been shut down; that many people had given up, gotten scared off, and gone back where they came from. Dad still wonders exactly how many people were lost in the confusion. At last count he figures that three hundred went off the Truehope radar because of that raid. Three hundred potential Deboras. He never stops talking about the loss, the damage. Not to Truehope, but to all those families who wouldn't find relief.

Not everyone was lost or fooled into diving back to the drugs. Individual smuggling efforts were working well enough to bring cases of product into Canada, and a friend-to-friend system of sharing had provided enough supplement for almost everyone who needed it. Dad and David went to court to settle the question of whether the search and seizure were legal. The judge allowed the agents to keep the stuff, to look through it for evidence, but he asked several questions. The raid may be legal, but is it ethical? This company sues you for what it deems an illegal seizure of product at the Canadian border, and you respond with a search on its property to go through the files—and you implement this raid using the very agents the company named in the suit? Is this ethical?

When is putting policy over people ever ethical?

46

Shawn said he'd get me on the stand after lunch. But first Sabine, another Red Umbrella friend, will finish her testimony. Another testimony I will not hear, not this time. But I have heard it before, on Parliament Hill, in front of the cameras, and broadcast on the radio via a telephone interview.

Shawn will enter the Red Umbrella Parliament Hill news conference tape as evidence. Evidence that Sabine, with all of the other women, made every effort to find a resolution to the EMPowerplus embargo. Evidence that we were there, on the Hill, begging for help and telling our story, warning of the consequences of sending us back to a broken system that had never worked to make us well.

I remember Sabine's testimony in our press conference. She spoke honestly, innocently. She was hopeful that by telling her story she would preserve her life and save others. This slender woman, blonde, frail, with bright blue clear eyes and a sweet smile, stood in her dress and sandals, adjusted the microphone, and clasped her hands over the podium.

"I was diagnosed with rapid cycling bipolar disorder and a second condition, obsessive compulsive disorder." She speaks perfect English with a soft French accent.

"I heard voices that were telling me that I should not be alive, I had no right to be alive, that everyone would be so much better off if I was not alive. To counteract the emotional pain, I caused myself physical pain. Many times I would smash my head into the wall until I would knock myself unconscious—or I would cut myself.

"It's a feeling that's very, very hard to describe, and if you've never felt that way, it might be hard to imagine, but it's a feeling of such intense anxiety and panic, where nothing feels real. You feel very isolated. You don't feel like you belong anywhere or that you have anything that's worth living for."

Sabine spent more than ten percent of her marriage in a hospital, living with strangers for months at a time. When she broke through her meds and escaped the hospital, the police brought her back. Then she became a model patient, taking all the medication, exactly as prescribed. She took drugs for the panic and drugs for the depression; drugs for the highs and for the lows and for the side-effects of the other drugs. Anti-psychotics, anti-convulsants; and she suffered cardiac disturbances. When she wasn't in hospital for her mind, she was in intensive care for her heart.

"The cardiologist said, 'These dosages are frightening, and I can't believe that you're alive on these dosages.' The reply of my psychiatrist was, 'This is the only way we know how to keep her alive, because that's the only way we can drug her enough to keep her calm enough to prevent her from killing herself.'"

She gained one hundred pounds and she became diabetic—taking five shots per day and oral medications of every kind. She had liver damage, yellow eyes, and half of her hair fell out on her pillow in clumps. It clogged the shower drain when her husband Darryl would force her from bed to take a shower. He fed her, too, while she wore a bib. Three kids were also being raised by this kind and patient, dedicated man, like Dad, like Dana. Sabine spent three years bedridden, twenty hours a day in bed. Her bones became brittle, and there was another drug for the brittle bones.

How well I remember what it felt like in my own life. Sabine was drugged and delusional, sleeping for days on end, then rising, only to fall out the door or down the stairs, stumbling in a thick dark stupor.

"I wondered; why did I wake up? Why didn't I just die in my sleep? I can't live another day having to feel like this. So it was just amazing when I heard about Truehope. I went to see my psychiatrist and told her about EMPowerplus, and she said, 'Oh, okay. That's the pig study.' And she said, 'Well, I think—I think you might as well try it. Nothing we've done is helping you, and the medications are making you very, very sick. You know, you don't have anything to lose. You have my blessing.'"

Sabine didn't get better all at once, but a few weeks into the treatment she started doing normal things, rising from bed, washing a few dishes, and having a shower. In a few months she was working a part-time job. Then she was offered a full-time job at the local veterinarian clinic. A few years later they promoted her and paid for her university education so she could get her certificate.

"I'm no longer diabetic, that's completely cleared up, I lost sixty of the one hundred pounds, I'm physically active, and I'm active as a volunteer in my community. I feel like my life is just beginning."

But Sabine and I both know that sane today can be sick tomorrow. The illness is our constant companion. Excessive stress, digestive upset—even a simple flu bug—and we become mildly symptomatic. Mess with our sleep for more than three consecutive nights and we get agitated; add stress and a lack of appetite and we get confused; add adrenaline and a sick stomach and we become mini-versions of our old bipolar selves. And we both know where it goes from there. That's why I'm here waiting, and that's why Sabine is in there testifying. She works and pays taxes and gives back to her community. She lives with her husband and her children in their dream home on a wooded acreage. She rides her horses. She is free, and she is telling her story to the court, and I am sitting out here supporting her with my thoughts and prayers. Sabine is standing, one more time, for Truehope.

And out here in this lobby I *am* feeling mildly symptomatic. My gut is grinding. I think they call this anxiety.

47

I'm still waiting, but not so patiently now that I know it is my turn next. Now that I know they are in there, behind those doors, already talking about my part in Truehope, displaying the events on Parliament Hill, watching me tell my story on the tape made from our Red Umbrella presentation in the Charles Lynch room. By now everything has been said. What's left to say? I worry that I'll get on the stand and look at the judge, and he'll think, Her again?

He will have just finished watching a tired, determined, pregnant version of me on tape, saying exactly what I am going to say now. I'll be a waste of time up there, repeating what has been said by so many others. I'll swear to tell only the truth. But what is the truth?

Today I must testify that I am sane. Normal, happy, healthy. Is it the truth? I haven't slept well for days, and I can barely stand to eat. I know it's not good for me and that I am pushing the limits of Dad's miracle. I'll take better care of myself as soon as this is over. And things will be normal soon. It's just the pressure of being here, watching helplessly from the sidelines, waiting, waiting, waiting. Being far away from my kids, wondering: Are they okay? Are they sleeping well at Grandma Stringam's house? Are they eating? But even normal moms miss their kids. Even a normal woman would feel the pressure today. Right?

I think of how many times I have visited the bathroom to check myself in the mirror. Only two times this morning. All within normal ranges. *No, I'm not slipping.* I open my notebook and read a paragraph of notes. *Yes, I'm all right.* I'm not confused. I'm just scared. Even normal women get scared before they testify. Right? Most people fear public speaking more than—

"Autumn Stringam?"

—death.

They are calling me in. I stand and feel the charge of adrenaline flush my body, my neck, and my cheeks. I gather my umbrella, my notebook, and my purse and follow the bailiff. I am supercharged as the crowd watches me make my way from the back to the front of the room. I reach Dana and flash a smile, trying not to look worried. He takes my things from me, and when I don't move to go on, he smiles and nods me toward the front.

My thoughts speed beyond dial-up, beyond high-speed. What do I say? I look to Shawn for a clue but his head is in a binder. Shawn, you didn't prepare me, you didn't tell me how this goes. A clue? Anyone? The clerk is over there adjusting papers on her desk. I steady myself, holding the rail as I step up from the wooden floor onto the carpeted platform in my high heels. Don't trip, just don't trip.

There's a microphone with a red light. What does that mean? And my desk runs into another taller desk to my left, so I follow the wood grain and find a body. Black robes over a white dress shirt, flushed cheeks, a thick moustache; grandfatherly hands shuffling papers. It's the judge.

One chance to say it with no mistakes. He won't believe me, it's all too unbelievable, names and dates and places, what year was it? What year is it now? They used to ask me that in hospital. They asked me the date and I knew it then, I always knew the date, but I don't know it now.

The agents think I'm crazy. Crazy, still a lunatic, and if I can't settle down, they'll know it for sure. They'll go back to Anne McLellan and tell her she was right and tell her I wasn't worth her time, and I was never worth saving anyway.

Shawn speaks and the judge speaks and they sound like mumbles through a garden hose and the air is thick and hot and I think I might pass out. And here is the clerk with the Bible and my hand is on it, and I have sworn to tell the truth. The panic doesn't leave, but the air clears, and I feel my feet wiggling in my shoes, and I feel wisps of my hair tickling my face, and I am back, present in the present once more.

I take my right hand from the Bible and my left from the air and hold the oak slab that divides me from Shawn and his lectern, his table spread thick and deep with legal-sized binders full of letters and timelines, exhibits and videotapes, and notes. I face him, but I look sideways once more to greet Judge Meagher. This time he is looking my way, and his kind eyes and carefully combed chestnut hair remind me of Dad's.

But I have heard tales this week of the judge's quick anger, his impatience with bureaucratic drivel on the stand, and I pray a quick one-liner that I will leave this stand in one piece.

Shawn is ready to give me a lead-in, and everyone in the audience is looking at the back of his head. He stands with one hand in his pocket, cool and aloof, steps in front of his lectern, and raises the curtain on my testimony . . .

"Okay. Your part of this Truehope story. Can you tell us your part?"

"Sure. Do you just want me to start with the very beginning?"

"You might as well."

Where is the beginning? Which one? That's a pretty open-ended question, Shawn. I clasp my hands and clench my bum, but I can't stop my legs from wobbling, so I look at the judge. *One second, please.* I kick off my shoes under the desk and plant my nylon-covered feet in the carpet. With my feet on the floor I feel stronger and ready to tell my story.

"When I was a young child, I had symptoms of illness. I remember getting in trouble . . . Mom said I could never listen . . ."

I am talking about kindergarten. Shawn's eyes go wide. I can almost hear him barking: Ack! No, that's not what I meant, not *that* close to the beginning, but I can't stop myself now that I have started, and I am saying way more than he wanted and more than anyone needed to hear. Any minute now the judge will yawn and slam his gavel and throw me out the door and my shoes after me. I've got to get to the point.

I am embarrassed standing here, fishing for words. I am Exhibit A, the first crazy woman allegedly gone normal, and I feel I am blowing the trial. If I go to pieces, so goes the evidence that EMPowerplus works.

Dad's head is down—I think he's praying. David isn't looking. Dana's expression is a non-expression. He's feeling this with me, a blank canvas for my terror. I see my fear reflected in his eyes, and he is on the edge of his seat. *Oh.*

I am hearing the words from my mouth. Oh dear, even I am bored by them. After Sabine's touching story, I am Autumn Ativan, putting them to sleep. I must figure out how to seem normal, not boring. It's harder than it might seem to look sane and talk about crazy.

Help me, please!

" . . . By the end of high school I couldn't even tell time on a conventional clock."

My prayer is answered through Shawn's mouth. "What do you mean?"

"Just a lot of confusion. A lot of racing thoughts . . . They were monitoring my art from art class. I still have one of my big paintings that the counsellor called me in to talk about, to ask about my thoughts. I guess it was pretty dark."

Focus on Shawn. Was that good? Yes, he's encouraging me by a twitch of his mouth, by a sharpening of his eye into a half-wink. More of that? Twitch. More of the weird stuff? Wink.

I jump into the teen years, mania, too many boyfriends, my marriage. My life sounds stranger than I imagined it would. As I expose it to the air of the courtroom, under oath, it does sound bizarre, even to me. No, worse than that. My words feel like projectile vomit. My life makes me sick. But not my audience. I can see that now. I can see that talking about sickness might even make me seem normal. Certainly when I was at my weirdest, I never admitted being ill.

So much private information spilling straight from my heart: "And I was pretty delusional right then, and I crashed . . ."

But my words don't reach the Health Canada agents. They just sit on their benches, thumbing their messages on BlackBerrys, doodling notes on pads of paper. They don't know me and they don't want to hear me. I am a waste of their time. They think I am a pawn in a game Dad is playing. They think I am a sob story to get Dad off that nasty $500 fine. I begin speaking to them so that they will pay attention.

"I couldn't keep a job."

"I couldn't function."

"I was paranoid and afraid all of the time."

"I had a lot of visions of stabbing through my belly and stabbing the baby and then bleeding out. I had it all planned out."

"Crazy flapping, scratching my face, the same movement over and over and over again, and I couldn't get it under control. It looked like this, first like this, then this, then I'd go over." I'm showing them, but they don't look for long.

"I got to the point where I would see little faces. They were pointy at the top and pointy at the bottom, and they would be in the mirror or a reflective glass . . ."

The Health Canada people don't care. They keep their heads down, keep thumbing messages to Ottawa, and I don't want to be telling the story at all. But I keep going. Pearls before swine, Dad would call it.

"Do you need a Kleenex, Ms. Stringam?" Shawn is in front of me.

I take the Kleenex and wipe my eyes, careful not to smear my mascara. I look up and lock eyes with Mr. Brown, Dad's prosecutor. He's sitting in his brown suit with his short thin fashion-forward tie. A pen in hand, but not taking notes. He's looking at me—at my eyes, and in that moment I know he knows the truth. Beyond him, though, beyond the wall, his employers sit, still thumbing messages, still averting their eyes from my gaze. I will give them something worth ignoring, something not pretty.

Don't do it.

Shawn nods and Mr. Brown shuffles and the judge is looking right at me.

Yes, I will do it, will say it, will humiliate myself. If they haven't seen the worst, how will they recognize the best?

I lay down whatever is left of my pride. "If I was alone, there were times when I actually had to go to the—use the kitchen sink as a toilet because I couldn't go into the bathroom. That's pretty low. That's pretty embarrassing." With that I give Shawn everything he never wanted to know about me, but everything that would prove the difference between me then and me now.

"I had to shower with my clothes on because the faces were all around me and they were talking to each other, saying if they could look in my eyes, they'd know the way to kill me. I tried to keep them from seeing that I was seeing them. I kept my eyes closed and called my sister. I just knew I wasn't going to make it through the day. That was the day I ended up in the psych ward for the first time."

Some of this I have never admitted to, and for good reason. Women like me don't have lives, husbands, babies. Women like me are beyond hope. I tell these details anyway. If people don't believe me now, it won't matter. And I'm way over being embarrassed about my illness.

I give what I have to, but I don't give them Mom. I can't. I decided it the moment I stepped onto the stand, when I realized my words were falling short of the agents' ears. I am horrified at my admissions, admissions of insanity given without the opportunity to explain, to justify, to soften. Words easily taken out of context. A telling that will follow me the rest of my life somewhere on public record. I told the truth, the whole truth, and nothing but the truth, and in so doing I could not protect myself from me. But I protected Mom. I gave all of me and none of Mom.

Now it's time to move on. The worst is over.

Shawn prompts.

"So, March 18th, 1996, what was your health like?"

That was the last day I took a psych drug. "If you'd asked me then, I'd have told you I was all better. When I look back now, I realize there's just been so much improvement over the years. Over the first year it was phenomenal improvement. You know, just not hallucinating, I thought that was as good as it could get. I didn't realize then that I was going to be able to read again, and tell time, and concentrate, and write."

I tell them about Dad and David's discovery, the relief, the restoration, how the hole in my chest closed up, how the illness went away, how my reflection in the mirror changed, how I overcame the habits of my illness.

"There was a little while, a transition time, after the medications, where, if I was faced with something that was really stressful, I would still flap, for lack of knowing what else to do, I think, and then I got to this place where I realized, 'Geez, you know, that's not okay any more,' so I had to figure out other ways to deal with stress, and all those habits have just kind of fallen off."

I tell them about living a new, normal life with Dana and my James. I tell them about having my girls, Samantha, Melanie, and Meagan.

"Okay. Do you need people to care for your children like you did when you were . . ."

"No, no. I'm a stay-at-home mom, and I'm a writer, and I help support other people who want to go through the same process that I went through, so I do mentoring, and I volunteer in my community. I do a lot of really normal things. I teach Sunday School."

I pause. The judge is listening, looking. Mr. Brown is watching. Shawn wants more. Go on, testify to the normal in you now.

"I just—I am involved in a full, normal life in a great marriage with a fantastic husband, with four great kids including a four-year-old and a two-year-old and a six-year-old. That's not really easy to deal with, but I'm doing it, and I love it. It's everything I ever wanted."

Shawn smiles and paces toward me. "Okay, so do you still spend the day in bed or anything?"

"Never." I laugh. "That would be a luxury." Judge Meagher chuckles and Shawn grins; the audience rustles and titters. "No. I get up with the rest of the world, and I function all day, plus some."

Having testified to my sanity, I begin my testimony about government intervention, the fear of having no legal access to the supplement:

"I got a letter saying that my product had been turned back at the border because it was illegal. So we chose to have the product sent stateside and then brought it across quietly. That's degrading. I'm an honest person. I really believe in obeying the laws of this country, and so it's degrading when you have to break the law and conspire to get vitamins and minerals, but I didn't have another option. If I can't get it, my only other option is to get sick. And that's just not a place I can go, not when I have four kids to care for. It's not a thing I want to put my husband through again. It's just—it's not an acceptable option for me to get sick again."

I look at the Health Canada agents. Did you think I wasn't worth saving? Well, here I am. If we met at the bowling alley, you'd see me with my son and you'd smile because he was happy and we are goofing, cheering, playing together. If you saw me at the dance studio with my three girls in tights and ponytails and little leather shoes, you'd grin because they look like me and I am gentle and they are bouncy, happy, smiley girls. But we aren't there, are we? We are here in this awful courtroom and you can't even look my way.

Shawn plays Dad's taped recording of me and Chantelle on the crisis line. The sound of her voice makes me sick for her. If anyone is a pawn . . .

Shawn has finished with me. "All right. Thank you, Ms. Stringam. Those are my questions. My friend might have some questions for you." Sabine got off without a cross-examination, but Mr. Brown stands and moves to the lectern.

Mr. Brown. I haven't thought of him as scary. He has been friendly, pleasant in the lobby, and kind in the elevator. But now he is talking fast and using his hand, fingers pinched together as if he's holding a tiny turkey baster, trying to emphasize his point without pointing, saying that the original supplement was not actually EMPowerplus, but a cobbled-together mixture of different supplements found on the market, taken in a combination designed by Dad and David.

I am baffled by his line of questioning because I'm sure that the prosecution must have covered this before when Dad was testifying.

"Why didn't you go back to the original mixture when you couldn't get EMPowerplus again?"

"Because a year into treatment, the liquid from the supplier became unstable. It wasn't working, and I went from taking two bottles a month to six, and that amount still wasn't holding me well enough. My understanding is that when the batches were tested, they weren't the same as the original. It wasn't good enough."

"But it worked originally, right?"

"Yes, but the original product wasn't available any more."

"Well, was it that you couldn't get it at all or that you didn't think it was as good as the original?"

I tell him again. It didn't work; it wasn't simply a matter of being picky or choosing Dad's supplement over another already available brand. The original product was not on the market any more. The original was a natural product, mined from organic material. It was inconsistent because the mine was different from dig to dig.

"Well," he chides, "it's interesting to me that you seemed to have great success with the original product, and then suddenly it's not useful when EMPowerplus becomes available."

He's playing games. I spell it out.

"The original product wasn't the same product any more. When the demand went up, the company switched mines. Everything changed, colour, taste. It was not the same product. In fact, we tried two other products before we found a manufacturer available for a stable product that actually worked without the ups and downs."

"So this stable mineral would have been available then."

More games. I put my hands on the top of the podium and look him in the eye. I tell him the stable mineral became available only when Dad and David created it. "The stable mineral being the all-in-one-product, EMPowerplus."

And with that, he's had enough. He thanks me and sits down, and I see it in his eyes. He didn't mean it. It's just his job. Prosecutors, Health Canada agents, they all have to have work.

I am excused. I slide back into my shoes and step down from the stand. I am composed on the outside, steaming on the inside.

I slide in and sit next to Dana, and he takes my hand tightly in his. I sit a moment and feel emotion wash over me. I miss Mom so much in this moment. She would have done a better job. She would have told her story, defended Dad, she would have ended Mr. Brown's questions faster and better—and she would have gone after him, too.

I sit as the court continues, but I block the proceedings out. I have an open-ended prayer to finish. *This would have been her moment, Lord. She would have done it better, and oh, how I wish she were here with me now.* Before I can say my *Amen*, I feel the answer. A wave of peace and a vision of Mom and me. We look happy together, understanding each other, opposite sides of a painted butterfly, beautiful and messy all at once. Her story has become mine, and my life has become, in some strange way, hers, and she knows it and I know. There is no way to separate us. I told her story when I told my own.

48

Yesterday was a day to endure, but today is the day to enjoy. Dr. Popper is coming; in fact, he arrived last night, flying in from Boston. He's here to stand for Dad and David, to stand for Truehope. I can barely contain my excitement.

Dana and I are up and out of our hotel bed early. He grabs a yogurt, and I hit the shower. Then he's in the shower, and I am tipping my head for a blow dry, zipping into my skirt. Rollers and lipstick and mascara do themselves in a whirlwind about my head, my hands flying as if I have extras. I am ready to go before Dana is even dried off.

"Whoa, someone is excited." Dana laughs, and I hurry him into his pants and shoes and shirt and tie. And I remember my vow to take care of myself. I swallow my EMPowerplus and grab a yogurt to eat on the way to the courthouse.

We battle rush-hour traffic, park in the icy lot across the road, and step through the slush, guarding our faces and holding our coats shut against the cruel fingers of the wind whipping and swirling in the canyons of downtown Calgary. The wind is in a hurry, and so am I.

I want to be there early enough to meet Dr. Popper before court begins. We step over gritty gutters and wait for the trains to pass. At long last we get past the subway tracks and step in from the cold. Waiting for the elevator, I smooth my hair and run my fingers under my eye makeup to wipe away wind-whipped tears.

"Do I look sane?"

Dana looks me over. "Do you think he'll think otherwise?"

"I don't know. Guys like him make me nervous. He'll be looking right through me, y'know."

"It's been a decade, babe. You have nothing to worry about." Dana kisses my head and scoots me onto the opening elevator.

"Are Dad and David here already?" I hope so.

"They were supposed to come in early with Shawn."

The elevator dings and bumps to a stop, and the doors glide open to expose an empty lobby. I am pleased to step into the courtroom once again, this time not to take the stand but to enjoy someone else's testimony. And they *are* here. Gathered at the front, beyond the wooden ledge dividing public from court, stand Dr. Bonnie Kaplan, Dad, David, Shawn Buckley, and our guest of honour. I know him before any introductions. At last.

I leave my purse and notepad on the bench and gather my courage to go to the group. Bonnie sees me coming and points him toward me.

"Charlie, have you met Autumn?"

"Oh, this is—so you are *the* Autumn? Oh, you *do* exist." He puts out his hand and grins.

"No—I mean yes, and you are Dr. Popper?"

"Oh, call me Charlie. I've heard so much about you, your story. Your dad told me about you the first time we met, so encouraging, so nice to put your face to the story. You. You really are well." And my guard drops completely.

"Yes, oh yes, I'm so good. I am so excited to finally meet you, I have been so grateful for the work you have done—are doing. You and Bonnie, I . . ."

"Oh no, it's Tony, David, they are the ones who deserve thanks." He looks at Dad and shoots a grin in his direction before turning to me again.

"Say, how long has it been now for you?"

"It's been a good decade, three daughters, and my son is well, he's almost fourteen. I stopped my last drugs ten years ago this week—four days from now, March 28th."

Bonnie steps in to vouch for me. She wants Charlie to know what she knows. "Really, Charlie, this girl is super. She's a mom and writing a book and teaching a class, right?"

She says it with pride; she's seen me change, seen me come a long way over the years. This almost feels like a high school reunion, celebrating a decade of being out of the institution. He's happy for me, and I'm happy to stand in this circle, with two very independent thinkers who know my history and yet, because of their own clinical experience, actually believe me when I say I am well.

"What class?" Dr. Popper probes.

"Oh, no big deal, it's adult Sunday school—Old Testament this year . . ."

"Tough subject, heavy reading." Dr. Popper is still searching me for clues. He's fascinated by this long-time user of the novel treatment that has brought us all—prosecutors, crazies, doctors, and normals—to this four-dimensional co-ordinate in God's universe.

"I'm still improving. Still getting better every year, I think." *No, I know.* "I know it's been a decade, but I swear, every year I notice new things, concentration, information absorption, things I never thought I'd ever get back. I'm healthy. I think better-than-average healthy."

"Yes, you are so clear. Your eyes. It's good to see you so well."

I am shaking my head, both embarrassed at the attention and relieved at the diagnosis. I'm holding Dana's hand and stunned that Dr. Popper is at least half as excited to meet me as I am to meet him.

"Let's get to our seats. Please. Take your seats, people." Shawn is calling to the packed courtroom before the judge and the clerk come in, and everyone scrambles. It's like a game of musical chairs.

This time Health Canada agents and Truehope supporters are outnumbered only by members of the press. Everyone wants to know why Dr. Popper would come all the way from Boston and what he could possibly say about Truehope. Dana and I squeeze in on the end of a row, packed thigh-to-thigh. I pull out my notebook. It's my turn. I want to study Dr. Popper, put him under my microscope. As I told the court yesterday, I'm a writer.

He's a lot like I expected, small frame, grey hair . . . fifty-something? Confident, clear, concise. I expected businesslike, aloof, perhaps condescending, and he is none of these; only humble and kind. And I see something in his eyes that I sometimes see in my son's eyes. A glint of mischief.

Judge Meagher arrives, and the clerk calls us to order. Shawn introduces Dr. Popper.

"Your Honour, Dr. Popper has a long history of teaching psychiatrists at Harvard Medical School. He doesn't teach the medical students, he teaches the psychiatrists. When other psychiatrists can't solve problems in children and adolescents, they get referred to him as a specialist among psychiatrists. I'm not just calling a psychiatrist as a witness. I am calling a psychiatrist who in the field of psychiatry is the leading expert in that area. And it will become germane to his evidence for trial."

Shawn reviews Dr. Popper's curriculum vitae, a testament to his education, his career, his specialties and accomplishments. I catch the highlights:

Educated at Princeton, then Harvard; he took three years away from the Harvard system to do research at the renowned National Institute of Mental Health. Then returned to Harvard to pioneer the child and adolescent psychopharmacology program at McLean Hospital, giving the first ever course for residents in child and adolescent psychiatry in the United States.

Developed courses and taught psychiatrists nationwide through the American Psychiatric Association; did similar work for the American Academy of Child and Adolescent Psychopharmacology. And he ran those programs for years.

Went on to run a more advanced study group for psychopharmacologists who are already well trained and advanced in their fields, wrote books, developed new treatment modalities for kids and teens, and took on a private practice for patients who were not responding to typical treatment. Acts as a consultant to other Harvard hospitals, including Children's Hospital and the Massachusetts Mental Health Center in Boston.

His reading glasses perched on his nose, looking over his notes as he speaks, Judge Meagher accepts Dr. Popper as an expert witness.

"I am satisfied on the review of Dr. Popper's curriculum vitae, his extensive experience, in fact pioneering in the field of child and adolescent psychiatry and psychopharmacology. He is qualified to give expert evidence in all areas of psychiatry, the diagnosis of mental illness, and with regards to the benefits and risks of different treatments for mental illnesses."

The court gives Dr. Popper a chair because his testimony will take a very long time, and he settles back to tell of his discovery of Truehope.

"I have for my entire career been very much the sort of mainstream child and adolescent psychopharmacology psychiatrist/physician who paid, frankly, next to no attention to nutritional factors, either in my professional life or in my personal life. It just was not an area that struck me as of interest." He goes on, describing a phone call he received just before Thanksgiving 2000 from a colleague, asking him to come and see a presentation by Dr. Bonnie Kaplan.

"So I told him, no thanks. It's a little strange. It's outside my field. I explained to him vitamins and minerals don't mean a whole lot to me. But thanks for calling and have a nice holiday."

Another colleague called and invited him again. Again he said no. Then a third call came. Finally, he agreed to go, booking two hours out of his day. He went to the meeting and heard from not only Dr. Kaplan, but also Dad and David.

Oh. This is the meeting that Dad told me about years ago, when I was pregnant with Melanie, when he was so excited. It had been such a success. I pat Dana's arm and jot a note to remind him of that conversation. But the meeting as described by Dr. Popper sounds very different from Dad's take on it.

"Tony and David described treating a lot of people, like, three thousand bipolar people, which is an enormous number of treatments. Bonnie had more scientific evidence, but it was far from perfect data, and it all struck me as very strange. I listened to them, and they made some claims about this treatment that struck me as pretty obviously ridiculous."

He counts the claims like strikes in a baseball game: "They said this treatment would effectively treat eighty percent of bipolar patients." He leans back and rolls his eyes. "Jeez, lithium, the best of treatments, only has a range of sixty-five or seventy percent response rate. There was certainly no theoretical reason to think that a treatment like that would work. There was nothing in psychiatry that was even looking in that general direction. So their claim of an eighty percent response rate struck me as bogus. False. They're amateurs. They're enthusiasts. Strike one.

"This is just what I was afraid I was going to hear when I said yes to this meeting," he adds, leaning forward to rest his elbows on the desk.

"A second claim, more ridiculous than the first, was that when they treated patients who were not previously on psychiatric medications with EMPowerplus, they could see a clinical improvement within five days. Five days? Nothing in psychiatry works that fast. At best, a week or two or three just to get to adequate blood levels, add five or ten days beyond that to see an improvement. Ridiculous. Obviously false. Strike two.

"There was one last claim, that adding this EMPowerplus stuff to somebody on a stable psychiatric regimen would amplify the effects of the drugs and make them so intolerably sick that they would be forced to lower the medication—even eliminate the medication altogether. Enough. Strike three and I am out of here."

Dr. Popper smiles and pushes back in his chair, his hands flat on the desk, as if he might actually go somewhere. He owns the room, plays his audience.

"What am I doing in this room? And I've been in this room for an hour and life is short. And I gotta get out of here."

Dana and I try hard to compose ourselves, to laugh in our hands, in our sleeves, but the courtroom is electric. We on the Truehope benches have all made those claims; most of us have lived them ourselves.

Popper needed to make his escape. So he lied. He told Dad and the others that he had an appointment at two. He said he'd like to think about it, read up on it. He asked for a list of ingredients, and they didn't have one, but David offered him a bottle of the supplement, pushed it on him, really.

"I said, 'No, no, no, no.' I knew that the bottle cost seventy-five dollars. I didn't want them wasting seventy-five dollars on me. 'Just e-mail me with the list,' I said. But David Hardy was pretty insistent. 'Just take the bottle, just take it, it's fine. We have plenty of them. Just take the bottle.' "

So Popper took it and said thanks and stuffed the bottle in his jacket. He was going to be walking through McLean Hospital, the most prestigious of all mental health hospitals, a learning hospital for Harvard University, and he could not be seen with a cheesy bottle of

EMPowerplus in hand. It had a label with a lighthouse and Truehope splashed all over it. Five minutes and he was back in his office. Now what? Where would he hide the bottle of pig pills?

He's twisting his face into embarrassed concern, remembering the scene. He's on stage, working the crowd.

The garbage? No, the cleaning lady might find it and pull it out, thinking he'd dropped it. She'd ask him what it was.

No. He'd hide it well behind a stack of medical journals where no parent, child, or cleaning lady would look and ask questions.

"Well, a really strange thing happened that day. It's very odd. That evening around five, I got a call from one of my child psychiatry colleagues who said, Could you please consult on my child as soon as possible, like, right now? And frankly, if it was anybody else, I'd say, 'Well, Jeez, you know I can certainly see you in a couple of months or three months,' something like that, but this was a colleague and a friend."

They came right over: the psychiatrist friend, his social-worker wife, and their ten-year-old out-of-control bipolar boy. Dr. Popper described how the child had tantrums for hours a day, every day, spinning on the floor out of control. Only bipolar disorder or cocaine would cause this kind of behaviour, and he knew the parents—it was not cocaine. He saw the child and did an evaluation to fill out the clinical picture.

He'd need to see the child a second time before starting a serious psychiatric medication. The parents knew Popper's reasoning but begged for a little mercy. The diagnosis was clear, the father was a psychiatrist himself, he knew what his son was dealing with. Couldn't they start now? Another week like this would be unbearable.

Dr. Popper needed another visit to get a full picture, and any drug would change that picture, mess up his reading of the symptoms. So what could he give them that was sure to do *nothing*, and still make them feel better about doing *something*?

Oh yes, that bottle stuffed behind the journals.

"So I said, 'Look, you know I heard about this really strange treatment today. These three Canadians came to tell us about this weird-sounding treatment."

He told them about the three strikes and was very clear about his attitude, but the parents said they still wanted to try it. So he pulled the bottle out from behind the journals and handed it to them.

"I was just thrilled to get it out of my office. Just delighted. I told them how to start, said I'd see them in a week. And I was perfectly satisfied that I was going to get a clean read on the kid."

Four days later the father called to say that the tantrums were gone. Not better, not even a lot better. Gone.

Dr. Popper thought it was a placebo effect, but it was very unusual to see a placebo effect of that magnitude in a child with daily two-to-four-hour-a-day temper tantrums. No vitamin or mineral could do that. No drug could do that. So the effect had to be placebo. Clear and simple.

But he told the parents, "Oh, that's wonderful," and invited them to come in again in three days. "I figured, in a few more days that placebo effect is going to wear off. I'll get my nice clean look at the kid and see what he's about." Seven days into the treatment the family arrived and the kid was "warm, thoughtful, intelligent. A totally different child . . . So I was floored and I said to myself, this is still a placebo."

He would see them again in another week.

Fourteen days passed and the child was bright, articulate, sensitive. Dr. Popper was baffled, and the parents had ordered a box of bottles from Truehope.

But the bottles did not arrive. Back in Alberta, Truehope was experiencing some growing pains, developing a new distribution program to avoid running into problems with Health Canada, and the new American shipping department was struggling with the Christmas rush. The little boy would have to go without before he ever really got started.

Starting and stopping the supplement in the early stages of recovery never works for anyone and certainly not for Dr. Popper's young patient. Forty-eight hours after the first bottle ran out, the tantrums were back full force. It was a complete reversal of symptoms. Dr. Popper offered conventional medication, but the parents said they'd wait for the Truehope package.

The boy had a tantrum every day for a week. The Truehope package still hadn't arrived, and the family was dreading a coming vacation. So Dr. Popper took a list of ingredients and went to the store.

"I frankly made a scene by buying a hundred bottles to try to get the various ingredients in the right forms and in the right proportion, to try to get a reasonable balance. I could get only twenty-eight of the thirty-six ingredients in the product, and the portions weren't a great match to the original, but it was an approximation."

Dr. Popper gave the bottles to the father and felt ridiculous doing it. He was just trying to help them through a tough time, restoring a little sanity for the family . . . and satisfying a little curiosity of his own.

"So they gave the kid this, you know, mess of pills. It was a huge number of pills. They went on their vacation and called me to say it wasn't like the original formula, but he was about sixty percent better than before. The vacation was workable. And that was the first time I began to believe that maybe there was something to this. Maybe. Because the ingredients I bought were off a store shelf, not some strange bottle arriving from elsewhere. I mean, who knows, they could have had Zyprexa, or lithium, or Thorazine in the pills that were being labeled EMPowerplus; I didn't know. But I knew what I bought was from a legitimate store and labelled properly, and they were getting sixty percent out of it. So it began to dawn on me that maybe this wasn't a placebo."

It dawns on us that Dr. Popper's skepticism, his reluctance to become a Truehope believer, was the best testimony that could ever be presented on our behalf. The crowd becomes still, listening to a masterpiece unfold. It's not funny any more; it's magic.

"They came back from their vacation. The package still hadn't arrived. He went back to school, and interestingly, the teachers said that he was about sixty percent better, entirely on their own. Then the package arrived, and the child went back on EMPowerplus, and the father called me four days later and said that the tantrums were gone, totally gone."

Dr. Popper can see the audience, see Mr. Brown at the prosecution table and the agents behind him, and he knows he has just told an incredible, ridiculous story. Still, he needs to explain, to put his observations into perspective. He now transforms from entertainer to teacher sitting forward in his chair.

"Now, that's actually pretty good evidence. That's the kind of thing we often do in clinical practice to try to prove that a treatment works. You apply a treatment, see an effect, withdraw or lower the dose or withdraw the treatment, see a return of symptoms, put back. In this case we had an intermediate product, then the original and a full response. So that's several reversals, and each reversal strengthens the case that there is a causal relationship between the drug treatment and the response. So that, at that point, was really extreme, strong evidence, and it really made me pay attention."

I watch Dr. Popper telling his story with confidence and humour. I see Dad and David sitting next to each other on the front bench, nodding and chuckling and listening so carefully.

Dr. Popper ends the telling of the boy's story with an epilogue. The boy grew into a teen and didn't like swallowing all those pills any more.

"He went on conventional medications, and he did not do badly with them. But they didn't work as well. He became chronically irritable . . . not like his old self—absolutely unmistakably not his old self. And he complained that the medicines made his mind foggy, that he couldn't think as clearly on the conventional medications."

He'd traded clarity of thought for swallowing.

"After six or eight months on conventional meds he decided he wanted to go back on EMPowerplus. The parents supported it. He made the transition back to EMPowerplus, and he's been fine ever since. No tantrums. He's not messing with the dose. And he is a superstar student."

Over the years Dr. Popper gave the option of this novel treatment to many of his patients, a hundred, maybe a hundred and fifty of them. In addition, he consulted with other physicians, who offered it to their patients, often when nothing else was working, three hundred to five hundred of them.

Off the top of his head he didn't really know the numbers, but this he did know: Those original strikes one, two, and three were not strikes after all. In his practice, his clinical experience, they had proven true. About eighty percent of his patients who tried EMPowerplus had a favourable response. An initial positive response on an unmedicated patient will occur, often within five days, and those who are medicated must be monitored very, very carefully as they make the transition from medication to EMPowerplus.

He beams as he retracts each strike, counting them back on his fingers.

He says the process is not simple; because there are so many variables, only one who understands the process should advise. Most psychiatrists wouldn't believe the reaction could be happening, let alone know what to do in the process, because everything about it is in opposition to what they know about psychiatric treatments and typical responses. It's all backward.

Shawn leads him for hours more, on and on through questions of protocol, determining what would happen to Popper's patients should the supplement ever become unavailable. He answers with perfect clarity, never relinquishing control of his audience.

"Would there be a return of symptoms? Definitely. Would they be problematic? Of course. There's no question that there would be depressions emerging. There would be suicides. There would be hospitalizations. There would be violent attacks, probably some jailings, and I wouldn't have a prayer of being able to manage it. I'd have to select a relatively small number to manage myself and just refer the rest for conventional treatment.

"I don't choose for my patients. I tell them EMPowerplus is an alternative. It's not established. It does not have the same kind of data behind it at all, and that—that matters because we don't have controlled data either on effectiveness or controlled data on safety, and it's going to be years before we really have adequate data of that sort. But I also say that I have had my own experiences. I describe what they are, and I let my patients decide for themselves. They really need to wrestle with the decision at this stage . . . There is nothing straightforward about that kind of decision."

Dr. Popper calls for more research. He wants specialized training for physicians, teaching them a new protocol for a treatment that would be backward by standard wisdom. He wants data. He is a pioneer, respected by his peers. With Dad and David and Dr. Bonnie Kaplan he is on the cutting edge of a breakthrough in modern psychiatry that is sure to change the face of mental illness not just on Parliament Hill, but the whole world over.

Just when I think I have heard enough to keep me grinning for days, Shawn asks the question of all questions.

"If you came down with bipolar, what would you do after you got over your panic?"

The courtroom goes silent. Mr. Brown sits up straight in his chair, bracing himself on the table, ready to stand. The agents stop thumbing, the press stop scribbling. The question, and the moment, hang in the air like powder after a gunshot. I can hear it ringing in my ears. The moment is magnified by utter silence, the very lack of breathing in the room.

Then Mr. Brown settles back down again in his chair. Judge Meagher looks at him. *What, you aren't objecting to that question?*

Brown answers the judge's look. "Well, sir, it is a little speculative, but I want to hear the answer to the question."

"So do I." Judge Meagher smiles. "But if Dr. Popper is not comfortable giving an answer, then . . ."

"I—let me think it through. I'm—I might decide I don't want to answer that, but let me, let me just think it through." Dr. Popper is sitting forward, and so are Dad and David and Dana. I see that Popper still owns the court, now more than ever, but this question has hit him where he lives. This is personal.

"Do you want to take a break?" Judge Meagher asks.

"So, I can get—no. No, I am just—Let me just—So, this is after I get over my reaction to getting the diagnosis?"

Too personal, even in make-believe.

"Mmm-hmm." Buckley stands still. A moment more and I watch as something comes over Dr. Popper like a wind of confidence, and he tosses caution to it. He breathes deeply, straightens his back, and takes on a demeanour that is bold and steady.

"I actually probably would choose EMPower. I know the trials aren't there, but I've seen it, and I think given the choice between committing myself to a lifetime of lesser stability and mental fogging I would first want to try EMPower."

I want to cheer and jump up and down and high-five Dana and smack my dad on the back and punch David in the biceps. I want to shout, Hooray for you, Dr. Popper, for saying the truth and sticking your neck way, way out there. And don't worry, Dr. Popper, your reputation is big enough to carry you and me and Dad and David and Bonnie for a long time. And Bonnie will prove you right. Her work will prove you are right, she'll get you that data. Thank God for Dr. Popper.

But this is court and not an arena, and so I just sit still and watch pure joy settle over Dad and David. I hear the pencils scrawling on the press bench behind me, shuffles and mumbles and sighs of relief from the staff on the bench beside Dana. *Oh yes.*

Above all, I feel Dana's hand squeezing mine. He smiles at me, and I know this one will go down in the Truehope Hall of Fame for amazing courtroom moments.

The high lasted for days. Every chance we got, we recounted our favourite parts.

I hear the kids in the kitchen, clanking around for breakfast bowls.

I am lying next to Dana, my arm on his chest, my head resting on his arm in what he calls our Hollywood Position. It's so good to be home, waking up in our own bed.

"It's taken all of the stigma out of it for me," I mumble.

"What has?"

"Popper's testimony. I just—if every doctor knew what he did, the world would be a safer place for us, and I'd never have to be afraid of disclosing my history again."

"That's coming, you know." He touches my hair with his free hand. "A few years from now and it will be common knowledge. All that truth revealed in that courtroom—people will hear it."

"Yeah. Especially if we win the case."

"I guess we'll know in four months."

"They're awake!" We've been found out. Melanie yells to the others, and before long our bed is hopping with three little wrestlers, taking on their daddy, laughing and tickling and screeching, and James is standing in the doorway grinning at the mayhem and asking if he can go to a matinee with his friends for a Saturday afternoon outing. Life's right back to my kind of normal. And I love it.

49

Judgment. It's an interesting concept: all of our freedom and all of our validation rest on one man's opinion, derived from three weeks of testimony and a superior understanding of Canadian law. Judgment. On the one hand, the judge could deny the defence and charge Truehope five hundred bucks and be done with it. But on the other hand, if he bought the argument of necessity, he'd be making a statement that went way beyond the DIN issue. He'd be commenting on our right to choose and on the necessity of the Truehope program. And so, this judgment matters.

Today in the courtroom, awaiting that judgment, I sit second from the end of the row, pressed close to Dana, my hand in his. And I'm steaming as I review the final arguments in my mind. In his final arguments Mr. Brown said that the judge could not allow a defence of necessity. It wasn't necessary to have Truehope when we could have gone to the store and cobbled together legitimate products the way Dr. Popper did for the boy. And he argued that allowing a Truehope necessity defence opened the doors for the likes of cocaine dealers, who, when forced to shut down their operations, leave many people panicked and desperate for their product, perhaps even suicidal.

Now Judge Meagher speaks, but I lose my focus and I float off. I watch the judge, my dad, David Hardy, the others in the court, people so full of feeling. They nod their heads, smiling, grim, or elated, as Judge Meagher recounts our history. They are in sync, as if the clerk is flashing cue cards to prompt their next emotion.

"There was expert evidence at trial that it would have been impossible for the defendants to obtain a drug identification number for the supplement."

Health Canada had been asking the impossible.

Our people nod, shift, and exhale. He is seeing our truth.

"Health Canada . . . issued directions to Canada Customs to stop all shipments of the supplement from the United States into Canada. There was panic and confusion amongst the participants in the Truehope Program. Health Canada's response was to set up a 1-800 crisis line on which callers were advised that they should go see a psychiatrist."

Judge Meagher turns red even as he says it his way, and our people scowl, fists tighten, heads bow and shake. The insult of sending healthy people back to that hell still stings.

I feel my own face pulling at the right places, a taut smile here, a grimace there, but I'm not feeling this as deeply as I ought to. I feel like a spectator at a stranger's accident.

I should feel like Jerry—the Truehope support-line operator beside me. She's blonde with long fingernails, a smoker's rasp, and an exuberant smile. She used to take so much medication. I wonder how she survived the treatments that nearly wrecked her heart, liver, kidneys, and pancreas. She has been better for years, using Dad's miracle.

The judge says, "The defendants were overwhelmingly compelled to disobey the DIN regulation in order to protect the health, safety, and well-being of the users of the supplement and the support program."

Jerry makes new fists and hisses, *Yes*. Then she breaks into gritty sobs and rummages in her bag for a tissue to wipe her tears. She wasn't prepared for the tears and can't find one, so Catherine passes one over to her.

I should feel more like Catherine.

Catherine—sandy-haired, middle-aged, bright eyes gleaming behind her reading glasses. She's been well for years. She was the first to see the demand of cease-and-desist from Health Canada as it came over the fax machine. Only two weeks into her Truehope employment, she had to decide whether this cause was worth the fight, the guilt that plagued her whenever Truehope was accused of breaking the law.

Judge Meagher explains the legality of an illegal act. "Everyone who undertakes to do an act is under a legal duty to do it, if an omission to do the act may be dangerous to life. The defendants could have been at risk of criminal prosecution if they had stopped providing the supplement."

Catherine touches her face and raises her eyes to the roof, praying thanks. She knows now that she made the right choice to stay with Truehope. No more guilt.

Except for me. I feel guilty because I don't cry with them.

I want to feel like Celeste, my sister. Little CC, now a beautiful, independent young adult—determined to help other people and ready to defend our dad at every turn. She has treated her own moods with the supplement since she found herself too close to the edge that Mom and I went over. Celeste knows a blessing when she's received one.

She sits behind Dad and off to the right, where she can keep her eye on his profile. She takes her cues from him, trying to understand the judge through Dad's reactions.

The judge says ". . . the defendants had no reasonable legal alternative and took all reasonable care to comply with the law. . . . I find the defendants not guilty."

Tears roll down Dad's face, and Celeste reacts in kind, putting her face in her hands, droplets of soft vindication leaking through her fingers and into her lap. Shawn Buckley thanks the judge, and Celeste straightens her back and sets her eyes back on Dad again, who is smiling. She brushes the long locks from the damp on her cheeks and beams relief and pure joy. Dad was right. Now the whole world will know it.

The crowd stands, the judge bows and leaves. The room breaks into cheers, even the media scrum.

I should rejoice. I thought I'd feel the way I felt after the first vote in Parliament. When I thought we had won something then, I jumped on the furniture and bounced off the walls in victory. But I don't now. I just don't.

I have always known Dad was right. Now a few more people will hear it today on the six o'clock news. I speak for the cameras, duck into my car with Dana, and we return to our normal lives. I don't even turn on the TV to watch the spin that evening. Maybe I am just tired.

Four weeks later, I am in my car alone, on my way to a publicity event. My cell phone rings. It's Dad. He knows I'm out of town. He wouldn't call unless . . .

"Hey, Autumn. Guess what. They appealed."

"What?"

"They had a month to appeal. This was the twenty-ninth day."

"On what grounds?"

"The letter says they figure the judge erred in his decision. No one really needs the supplement. There are other options."

"How can they? Dad, they haven't got a leg to stand on."

"Ahhh, they're just playing the game."

I can't even speak.

"They're just buying time, honey, stalling the inquiry. Don't worry about it. I just thought you'd like to know."

"Yeah, thanks, Dad." I feel sick at heart. I know now: This is why I felt empty after trial. "I'll call you after I'm done here."

"Hey, Autumn. You think you'll help some people tonight?"

"Hope so."

"You'll be great. You have a great night. Love ya."

"Love ya, too, Dad."

Judge Meagher had been kind in his ruling, giving Shawn the defence of necessity but stopping just short of declaring the Health Canada treatment of Truehope an abuse of process. Shawn did not agree. He said it was absolutely an abuse of process. But he had to let it go.

Health Canada kept their Type Two Risk warning about EMPowerplus up on their website as a beacon to point to when the press came calling. And just when the press coverage was really picking up, and Dad and David and Shawn were in Ottawa asking for a ministerial inquiry into the actions of TPD Health Canada, the TPD agents found a new answer for the press. *We are appealing the judge's decision.* Of course, that announcement shut down the press; no one has won anything if the decision is under appeal.

Health Canada didn't really mean it, though. There was no appeal. It was merely a tactic to end the questions. Lessen the exposure. Once the press cooled off, they quietly took it back. Upon further review we have decided not to appeal.

50

I'm sitting in a hotel, typing out the final pages of my life thus far, and I am stumped. Only Dad can inspire me now. I dial his number and he answers.

"Hello." It's late and he's driving.

"Dad, do you have a minute?"

"Oh, hi, Autumn. What are you doing?"

"Just writing, working out the ending of this book. A garden would have been easier, Dad. A garden would have been poetic, but all I have is this mess of court and appeals, and I can't decide if we've won yet. Have we won?"

"Are you kidding?"

"No. Spell it out for me, Dad. Tell me what we have won. Every time I think it's over, it's just beginning, and I don't know if I can call that winning."

"Listen up, kiddo, let me tell you about what we have won." And he takes on a voice like a preacher's, and I picture him so many years ago when his hair was thick and brown: He's standing in his black dress pants and his white shirt and tie at the pulpit in Fort McMurray, a layman and volunteer clergyman, commanding the faith of his little flock of two hundred.

"We are selling the product legally, providing it to customers legally, helping people through our program legally, and that was happening years before the court case happened.

"We have exposed Health Canada and its abuse of its authority, and its agents will think twice before they put policy over people again, Autumn. They will think twice."

He's on a roll instantly, and I am scrawling his words as fast as my pen will fly.

"We have won a new respect for the mentally ill. They are no longer hopeless if they find Truehope. They are no longer stigmatized if they go on to live a life like the one you are living now.

"We won your life, Autumn, and Joe's life, and your kids' lives, and all of the family's. We won because, at the end of the day, I can protect my family—what's left of it—I can protect them from ever going to that hell again. Liberty, Autumn, we won liberty for the captives! Are you trapped any more? No. Are you afraid any more? No."

I can hear him pounding his steering wheel the way he used to thump the pulpit, before Mom died, before his life was changed forever. And it brings tears to my eyes.

"We won a battle that we never even wanted to fight, and there has been a power behind this that goes way beyond our abilities. We won before the fight even started because this victory isn't mine and it isn't David's. It's an answer to prayer, Autumn. It's a miracle. It's a miracle.

"We have won the right for you to choose to be well, to help as many people as you want to, to help them find their way out of the darkness of mental illness.

"Autumn, Bonnie Kaplan said it years ago, and I believe it. This may be the most significant breakthrough in mental health since the beginning of time, and we have won the right to use it and to share it. And oh, I wish your mother was here to see it. To be blessed by it the way you are. Aww. . . I miss her."

In the end, for Dad, it is always about her. I love that about him. And I have been blessed. So blessed.

This they can never take from me. A father who has loved me enough to fight to save me, to protect me, to save and protect others from my mother's fate. How I love him for his courage, his willing heart, and his stony determination to win a battle with no end in sight, and perhaps no earthly reward in store.

As for Dad, I think there is only one reward he truly seeks and that is to know that his beautiful Debora's life has meaning to others, to all those who become free of her illness with Truehope.

Being free of my mother's illness makes me different; I am Autumn and not Debora. I am still a part of her just the same. And I celebrate our similar paths as I find the blessings in our common experience. I thank God for that special moment, long ago, when Mom gave me a gift, a vision—the last tool I would need to forgive, to move on, to remember and rejoice without regret. She showed me a memory I had left somewhere in the back of my mind. A memory of painted wings.

In kindergarten I made folded paintings that turned into butterflies. Painting one side first, then folding the wet paint against the clean side of the paper, creating a mirror image. The first image was fresh and dark, while the second was muted, softer, but a mirror image just the same. A pair of wings. My mother and I.

When I look at my life, I see moments in those butterfly wings, moments tying my life to my mother's experience. Because of those wings, I find her in me. My adult path of loss and illness allows me to step back into my childhood to see her with new understanding.

She was in many ways a child, too, when she lost her father to suicide. Her grief made her an adult. She was a loving daughter, so consumed with his death, so desperate to set right the wrongs of his passing. She needed her dad, and she felt betrayed, abandoned, when he left her, starting her on her own path to suicide. She was unable to express this agony because she would not bring embarrassment to her family. She would not air their dirty laundry for the neighbours.

Forced to conceal her pain and to call his death an accident, a heart attack, she surely felt her own heart stop—stop loving, stop living. She kept the secret from us, all the while knowing that his secret was her destiny. And this knowledge consumed her.

There is kinship in these painted wings. She knew my pain before I understood hers. I am decorated in her agony, refined in my own, and I love her better for having been the muted side of the butterfly.

Some people say they see the hand of God in their lives. Mom saw His foot. She touched His wounds. A humble, tearful girl with a broken heart and burning fingers, clinging to a promise that, in the end, things would be all right; that in the end, justice would prevail, and she would be with Him. She is with Him. And I am free.

I see it now.

Because Debora took her own life, she saved mine. Her suicide set in motion the entire chain of events that rescued Joe and me. But it's not just a brother and a sister who will live because she died. Thousands, perhaps millions of other people, either those mentally ill or the loved ones of the mentally ill, will be spared some measure of grief. Few of those millions will know the part she played in their lives. Few will even know her name. But I will.

We still weep for her. So much of our everyday life is still about her. Every joy, every pain, every triumph is marked with the sting of her absence. Nearly thirteen years after her death, Dad finally came to a place of healing, some kind of closure, and set a proper stone on her grave. He said it took him that long to find the words to say goodbye to his dearest love. And he found the words in a testament of her faith, in a poem I wrote for her. He had the words engraved on her large pink stone.

His promise He keeps
He comes
With winds of redress
Cool and easy

Ashes scatter
In His presence
He lifts, we rise
To glorify Him

He brings the promised gift
And we are free
Beauty for Ashes.

AFTERWORD BY DR. CHARLES POPPER

Autumn Stringam's moving and unromanticized story rivets our attention on one of the countless human tragedies wrought by bipolar disorder. Autumn's triumph over her mind-straining circumstances involved extraordinary luck, coupled with her own determination and the fearlessness of the people closest to her, who created a daring new approach to treating mental illness.

Autumn's enthusiasm for her treatment is justified. By all accounts, EMPowerplus changed her life more profoundly than conventional medication treatments could. The success in her case is undeniable. And there are thousands more like her.

But it would be a mistake to infer from her good fortune that vitamin-mineral treatment would have a similar effect for all people with bipolar disorder. Treatments can work brilliantly for certain individuals but not at all for others.

There is an old joke in medicine that newly introduced treatments seem to work best when used quickly, before their side effects and limitations become known. This facetious and ironic saying highlights the fragility of scientific knowledge regarding new treatments and the need to maintain extreme caution in the face of "miraculous" cures; a new lover may seem perfect for the first few weeks or months, but a deeper and wiser love becomes possible only with the perspective gained through time and experience.

The only way to know whether a vitamin-mineral approach is effective for people with bipolar disorder generally is by conducting a series of large-scale, scientifically rigorous clinical trials. To date, we do not have even one such study.

Without large-scale controlled studies, we do not know whether Autumn's success would be experienced by 10% or 70% of people with bipolar disorder. We cannot know whether Autumn's response was due to the ingredients of EMPowerplus or due to psychological, situational, accidental, or random factors. And we cannot assess the side effects and the potential risks of EMPowerplus. While many people assume that vitamins and minerals are safe, these micronutrients can have serious toxic effects if employed improperly. Again, this makes it essential to have controlled trials of EMPowerplus, so that questions of safety as well as effectiveness can be clarified.

Controlled scientific studies of EMPowerplus are in the works, but it will take years before the results are in. At this point, individuals and families whose lives have been ravaged by bipolar disorder should exercise caution and balance in reacting to the initial observations on this seemingly promising approach. The initial findings are particularly challenging to physicians, because they do not fit easily into current psychiatric knowledge or theory on bipolar disorder. For patients and physicians alike, it would be a mistake to enthusiastically rush to use this treatment, and it would be a mistake to off-handedly dismiss it.

While waiting for controlled trials, it is critical for patients and families to know that there are well-established medical treatments for bipolar disorder. Although psychiatric medications did not work well for Autumn, they are life-giving and life-saving for the majority of people with bipolar disorder. Mood stabilizers, antidepressants, and antipsychotic medications are critical for the mental stability and well-being of many patients with mood disorders. Thousands of people with these conditions have been carefully studied under controlled scientific circumstances to support this claim. Because of that abundant evidence, these "established" treatments constitute the "standard of care" for treatment of bipolar disorder.

In my own clinical practice, I have seen encouraging effects of the micronutrient treatment in some cases, but I caution my patients that this is a new and unproven treatment whose safety and effectiveness have not been adequately evaluated.

Although the vitamin-mineral treatment can be viewed as an alternative to conventional psychiatric medications, it is probably more helpful to think of it as complementary. I have seen patients for whom EMPowerplus is better than conventional medications, and I have seen patients for whom conventional medications are better than EMPowerplus. And I have seen people for whom a combination of micronutrients and conventional medications produces a better clinical outcome than either approach alone. So there is nothing contradictory about medical and nutritional approaches. In fact, to view these approaches as "opposite camps" is anti-scientific; it reduces our ability to see that the larger goal is the service of patients with bipolar disorder, not the triumph of one idea over another.

EMPowerplus, at this early stage of investigation, is a single formula that is applied to all comers. If this approach proves encouraging, it is likely that this one-size-fits-all product will eventually be refined and tailored to the specific requirements of individual patients. Judging from everything we know in psychiatry, medicine, and biology, it would be a spectacular surprise if one formula or product was the optimal treatment for everyone.

Many clinicians who have been using EMPowerplus in their practices have already found variations on the original EMPowerplus formula that appear to enhance its effectiveness for specific individuals. In fact, Truehope has been changing the recipe for EMPowerplus over the years as it learns how to improve its overall usefulness in treating bipolar disorder and depression.

Mood disorders are far too dangerous, too diverse, and too complex to be managed by pills alone. Suicidality, aggressive violence, loss of hope, impulsive behaviour, impaired cause-and-effect judgment, and lack of self-protective intuitions should not be managed by self-help. Counselling, psychotherapy, family-oriented interventions, social skill training, development of coping skills, support programs, and community agencies can help. There is a need for a systematic restoration of judgment and perspective, a building of the ability to understand and think rationally about an illness that impairs judgment and feelings, and a reconstruction (or construction) of a reality-grounded self-esteem.

These are not supplied by pills and never will be. Patients and families need to learn how to seek help when needed, to understand this illness, to recognize early warning signs of recurrent symptoms, and to routinely take precautionary measures to reduce the risk of a return of symptoms.

To understand the illness, patients and families can learn to see that strengths as well as weaknesses are a part of bipolar disorder. Contrary to some stereotypes, many people with bipolar disorder have extraordinary strengths, especially in the realms of creativity, persistence and determination, generosity and altruism, and interpersonal sensitivity. Rather than viewing bipolar disorder as simply a medical illness, it may be more accurate to view it as a medical "condition"—and as part of the human condition—entailing both strengths and weaknesses. Helping people with bipolar conditions view their strengths as well as their weaknesses can help them view themselves and their conditions more fully and more accurately.

Certain people find it difficult to accept help, especially for something as personal and shameful as bipolar conditions can feel. Autumn had the advantage of many helpful and determined people around her. The most important thing that you can do to help a person with bipolar disorder is to help them seek treatment, especially at times when they need but do not want treatment. You can also help by showing that you do not blame them for their condition, by helping them use their opportunities and strengths, and by contributing money to support scientific research to develop new and better treatments.

For this remarkable story, we can thank Tony Stephan and David Hardy, the originators of the vitamin-mineral treatment, as well as Autumn and her brother Joe as its first beneficiaries. Stephan and Hardy showed courage and steadfastness in pursuing the development of this treatment, even in the face of legal obstacles, and in pressing for controlled clinical trials. Scientific studies on EMPowerplus are beginning to be conducted, especially through the efforts of Dr. Bonnie Kaplan at the University of Calgary in Alberta. So some day, we will know whether their excitement and efforts will have paid off. I'm betting that the clinical trials will become the foundation for an important new direction in psychiatric research, but one person's opinion is not what science is about. In the meantime, we watch with patience, and a balance of skepticism and hope.

Autumn's story is much larger than the amazing personal, medical, and political events she describes. Autumn makes each of us grapple with our own presence on earth and what we do with our lives. Whether the vitamin-mineral approach to treating mood conditions will ultimately be found to be scientifically sound is an open question. But regardless of the outcome of the research, Autumn and the people who have supported her have conveyed to us their hope—hope that new treatments can be found, hope that tragedy can be made temporary, hope that we can work together to make new things happen, and hope that our lives can have impact despite the odds.

—Charles Popper, M.D.
Harvard Medical School
August 2007

ACKNOWLEDGEMENTS

Mom, thanks for my life. It is the best gift to be the other side of your butterfly. Dad, thank you for my second life. You are the very definition of triumph over trial. Dana, your love, compassion, and patience are a miracle, and you are my Love Only. James, you are strength, integrity, and forgiveness. I am blessed to be your mom. Samantha, when God gave you to me, he traded beauty for ashes. You are beautiful. Melanie, you are pure evidence of God's love. You are sunshine and sparkles. Meagan, your determined, beautiful soul is the perfect reflection of my red umbrella. Angie and Sunni, thanks for being my closest companions through the darkest hours. David Hardy, you have brought validation to a miracle. Thanks for your quiet wisdom. James V. Smith, my mentor in writing, your teaching brought out the best in me. Thanks for your understanding and insight as I dragged you through the pages of my life! Sabine, Sheila, Suzanne, Deb O., Kristy, Debra C., Lu, and Patricia—my Red Umbrella friends—thanks for your friendship and courage. Life is too short to ever take a step backward! Sharon Unger, my friend in Shinah, may our efforts bless the lives of women everywhere, heal hearts, and strengthen families. Thank you for sharing the vision. Sheila Stanley, they say success is all about who you know . . . apparently, you are the person to know! Thank you for being a dear friend. Lee Davis Creal, my agent and friend, thank you for seeing my painted wings and stepping up with brilliance and energy to help bring my message to the world.

To the HarperCollins team, Noelle Zitzer, Sharon Kish, Lloyd Kelly, and Iris Tupholme, thank you for seeing the hope in my story and working so hard to let me tell it. To Alan Jones, thanks for the beautiful cover design. Special thanks to Brad Wilson, my trusted Collins editor, for taking the time to respect my story through the editorial process; you are talented and insightful, and your vision for bringing hope to the telling was pure inspiration. To Barbara Bower, my publicist, thank you for your enthusiasm and friendship. I couldn't ask for better representation. To Leo MacDonald, vice president of sales and champion of hope behind the scenes, thank you for giving me a chance to prove my sanity.

To David Kent, president of HarperCollins Canada, thank you for your commitment to do well and do good at the same time.

RESOURCES

Shinah House
P.O. Box 2587
Cardston, AB
T0K 0K0
Canada
(403) 653-7579
www.shinahhouse.org

Shinah House provides transitional housing and life-skills mentoring for persons recovering from mental illness. It is the place for all those struggling with mental illness to go, learn, grow, and become well.

All of Autumn Stringam's royalties from *A Promise of Hope* will be dedicated to the building of the first Shinah House in southern Alberta and the establishment of Shinah House concepts in many existing transitional homes across Canada.

Truehope Nutritional Support Ltd.
P.O. Box 888
Raymond, AB
T0K 2S0
Canada
(888) 878-3467
www.truehope.com

Truehope Nutritional Support Ltd. provides written and telephone resources that support mental and physical well-being in EMPowerplus users. Truehope also provides information and help to health care practitioners who are utilizing the Truehope nutritional protocol within their practices.

TrueHope Institute
234 Main Street
Shelby, MT
59474
USA
(800) 511-5156
www.truehopeinstitute.org

TrueHope Institute is a U.S.-registered non-profit charity [501(c)3] established to provide relief to those who suffer with mental illness through new and innovative mental health research, transitional housing and support programs, and treatment assistance programs for the indigent.

Canadian Mental Health Association, National Office
Phenix Professional Building
595 Montreal Road, Suite 303
Ottawa, ON
K1K 4L2
Canada
(613) 745-7750
www.cmha.ca

The Canadian Mental Health Association is a nation-wide charitable organization that promotes the mental health of all and supports the resilience and recovery of people experiencing mental illness.

National Institute of Mental Health
Public Information and Communications Branch
6001 Executive Boulevard, Room 8184, MSC 9663
Bethesda, MD
20892-9663
USA
(866) 615-6464
www.nimh.nih.gov

The National Institute of Mental Health's mission is to reduce the burden of mental illness and behavioural disorders through research on mind, brain, and behaviour. The current published studies on EMPowerplus can be found on the NIMH website.

The Organization for Bipolar Affective Disorder (OBAD)
1019 - 7th Ave SW
Calgary, AB
T2P 1A8
Canada
(866) 263-7408
www.obad.ca

OBAD helps people affected directly or indirectly by bipolar disorder, depression, and anxiety to live better lives. It offers internet links, resources, and peer support meetings.

Centre for Addiction and Mental Health
1001 Queen Street West
Toronto, ON
M6J 1H4
Canada
(416) 535-8501
www.camh.net

The Centre for Addiction and Mental Health provides links to many resources, including resources on bipolar disorder, information for parents who are looking to better understand how to manage drug education at home, background information on mental illness and addiction, and where to find regional resources in Ontario and beyond.

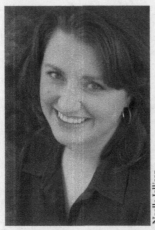

Noelle Jellison

AUTUMN STRINGAM was diagnosed with bipolar disorder when she was twenty and has been symptom-free for over ten years. As a public speaker, author of mental health resources and political advocate for the mentally ill, she has spread the hope of recovery to thousands of Canadians and a growing worldwide audience. Autumn Stringam lives in Idaho, with her husband and four children.